CHOLESTASIS

Edited by **Valeria Tripodi**
and **Silvia Lucagioli**

Cholestasis
Edited by Valeria Tripodi and Silvia Lucagioli

Published by InTech
Janeza Trdine 9, 51000 Rijeka, Croatia

Publishing Process Manager Irena Voric

Technical Editor Teodora Smiljanic

Cover Designer InTech Design Team

Additional hard copies can be obtained from orders@intechopen.com

Cholestasis, Edited by Valeria Tripodi and Silvia Lucagioli
p. cm.
ISBN 978-953-51-0043-0

For EU product safety concerns:
IN TECH d.o.o., Prolaz Marije Krucifikse Kozulić 3, 51000 Rijeka, Croatia,
info@intechopen.com or visit our website at intechopen.com.

Meet the editors

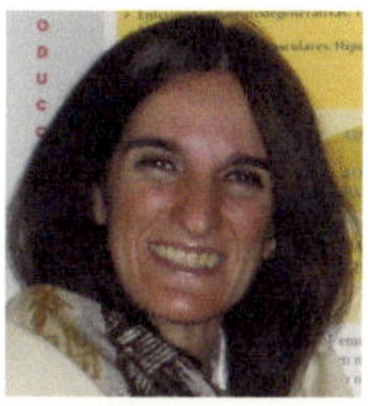

Dr Valeria Tripodi is Professor in the Faculty of Pharmacy and Biochemistry at the University of Buenos Aires and Investigator of the National Science Research Council (CONICET). She received a Biochemist degree from the University of Buenos Aires in 1992, a Master of Molecular Biology and Genetic Engineering in 1999, PhD in Clinical Biochemical in 2003, and she is a Licensed Teacher of the Teaching Career of University of Buenos Aires since 2008. Her main research is focused in the development of micro and nanoanalytical methodologies applied to diagnosis of different pathologies and pharmaceutical quality control. Under a multidisciplinary conception of the research, her group undertakes collaborative projects with research medical, and biopharmaceutical groups in Argentina. She supervises two doctoral theses and three fellows. Dr Tripodi is the author of more than 30 scientific articles and book chapters. She serves in the Editorial Board and as a permanent reviewer of several analytical and medical journals. She has recently founded the Analytical and Technological Laboratory of Clinical and Pharmaceutical Research.

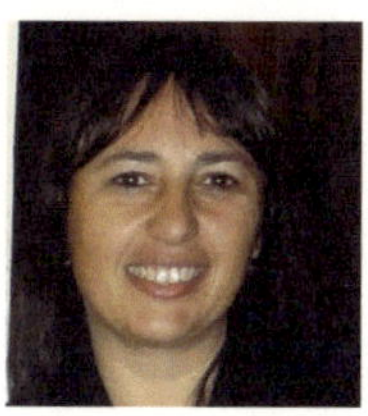

Dr Silvia Lucangioli is Associate Professor of the Pharmaceutical Technology Department at the Faculty of the Pharmacy and Biochemistry, University of Buenos Aires and Investigator of the National Science Research Council (CONICET). She received her Graduation in Pharmacy (1989), Licensure in Biochemistry-Pharmaceutical Industries (1991), PhD in Analytical Chemistry (2003) at the University of Buenos Aires, and she is a licensed teacher at the Teaching Career of University of Buenos Aires (2005). Her main research is focused on the development of analytical methodologies, including capillary electrophoresis based on electrokinetic chromatography, and microHPLC, applied in pharmaceutical and biopharmaceutical analysis. She supervises four doctoral theses, and two students. She has published over 30 scientific articles and book chapters. Dr Silvia Lucangioli has recently co-founded the Analytical and Technological Laboratory of Clinical and Pharmaceutical Research.

Contents

Preface

The aim of this book is the study of cholestasis from different points of view. Cholestasis is one of the most common and devastating manifestations of hereditary and acquired liver diseases. Since the importance of the disease has been made aware, there have been many research works, providing an increase of information. Identification of the molecular defect in cholestasis is not only important for diagnostic reasons, but also to emphasize that impaired transporter function has pathological consequences. Indeed, it is now becoming clear that impaired or down regulated transporter function is also involved in the pathogenesis of acquired cholestatic syndrome.

Linked to the diagnosis of cholestasis, an important area to study is the serum bile acid profiles. In this sense, a great development of analytical methodologies has allowed the relationship between them and the different types of cholestasis to be studied. The proper interpretation of serum bile acid profiles provides medical management against the disease.

Different models of induction of cholestasis have been designed in order to deepen understanding and clarify protective mechanisms, which could contribute to improved treatment of the pathology.

The complete understanding of cholestasis will provide an efficient treatment and an overall improvement in the patient life quality.

Dr. Valeria Tripodi and **Dr. Silvia Lucagioli**
Faculty of Pharmacy and Biochemistry,
University of Buenos Aires,
Argentina

Part 1

Medical Management

1

Intrahepatic Cholestasis of Pregnancy: The Usefulness of Serum Bile Acid Profile for Diagnosis and Treatment

Silvia Lucangioli[1,2] and Valeria Tripodi[2,3,*]
[1] *Department of Pharmaceutical Technology, Faculty of Pharmacy and Biochemistry, University of Buenos Aires, Buenos Aires,*
[2] *Consejo Nacional de Investigaciones Científicas y Tecnológicas, CONICET,*
[3] *Department of Analytical Chemistry and Physicochemistry, Faculty of Pharmacy and Biochemistry, University of Buenos Aires, Buenos Aires, Argentina*

1. Introduction

Intrahepatitic cholestasis of pregnancy (ICP), also called obstetric cholestasis, is a specific liver disease that takes place in the second or third trimester of gestation and spontaneously disappears after delivery (Shaw et al., 1982; Brites et al., 1998). Firstly reported by Ahfiled in 1883, it was after 1950 that the disease began to be considered of significance when several clinical cases were studied. It has lastly been highlighted the association of ICP with perinatal mortality and morbidity of newborns from cholestatic mothers (Pradhan, 2002). For pregnant women with cholestasis, quality of life can be impaired by itching, jaundice and fat malabsorption, but the prognosis of the mother is good. However, ICP is a condition with possible lethal outcome if it is not handled with care. Therefore, an early and accurate diagnosis of a risky pregnancy produced by ICP together with a safe medical treatment are essential to improve fetal outcome. (Diaferia et al., 1996; Bacq et al., 1995; Meng et al., 1997; Milkiewicz et al. 2002).

Puritus is usually the chief complaint and generally starts in the palms and soles, progressing to the arms and legs and eventually involves the trunk and face. There is additional progression from occasional to constant pruritus which can lead to sleep deprivation and irritability. Jaundice occurs in approximately 17-75% of ICP cases and telangiectasia and palmar erythema may be present in up to 60% of clinical cases (Mullaly et al.2001). It was found a weak correlation between bile acid levels and pruritus suggesting that the subjective symptom cannot be taken to predict severity of the disease. (Glantz et al., 2004)

Although it is an interesting matter, severity of maternal signs and symptoms does not seem to correlate with fetal prognosis and many obstetric clinics still choose to manage ICP pregnancies with expectance. Maternal monitoring of fetal movement has been described as normal until a few hours before delivery in cases of subsequent fetal demise.

---

* Corresponding Author

The prevalence of pregnancy cholestasis varies throughout the word being South America, specially Chile, the geographical area of higher percentage (12-22%) (Pradhan, 2002).

The exact pathogenesis of ICP is still unknown being probably of multifactorial causes. Genetic studies revealed a positive family history in 33-50 %, the condition is known to repeat in 40-70% of pregnancies and it is reported an endemic occurrence showing that a genetic factor should be taken into account (Lammert et al., 2000).

Levels of estrogens could also be involved in the development of ICP. This theory is based on the observations that the most common date of presentation of ICP is the third trimester of pregnancy when the estrogen levels are highest and is resolved promptly after delivery when placental hormones return to their normal levels. On the other hand, obstetric cholestasis resembles a similar condition that some women develop while taking oral contraceptive pills containing estrogens in the formulation. Moreover, twin pregnancies bothly display a higher incidence of ICP and more pronounced rises in estrogen levels (Pradham, 2002; Lammert et al., 2000).

In the pathogenesis of ICP, progesterone and its metabolites seem to play an even more important role than estrogens. It is described in the literature the development of ICP related symptoms after the administration of progesterone in a woman with a history of ICP (Lutz et al., 1969; Mullaly et al., 2001). It was also demonstrated that the profile of progesterone metabolites in plasma from patients with ICP is markedly different from the profile observed in normal pregnants (Sjövall et al, 1970, Laatikainen et a. 1974; Pascual et al. 2002).

Though the pathogenesis of the fetal death in ICP is not fully understood, the action of bile acids is strongly suspected to be implicated in mortality. During ICP there are a high bile acid levels in ammiotic fluid, cord plasma and meconium increasing the flux of bile acids from mother to fetus (Lammert et al., 2000). In cases of intrauterine fetal loss, observation of fetus autopsy is consistent with death from acute intrauterine anoxia. Meconium and bile acids, especially cholic acid (CA), have been indicated to induce vasoconstriction of human placental chorionic veins in vitro (Serrano et al., 1998) as well as to cause acute umbilical vein constriction (Altshuler et al., 1989; Altshuler et al., 1992). Although bile acid mechanisms are not yet defined, it is well known their toxic action. Thus, there is some experimental evidence that bile acids are involved in the mechanisms triggering fetal asphyxia in pregnancies complicated with ICP (Brites, 2002). It was also demonstrated that taurocholic acid (TCA), a bile acid increased in ICP, causes a decrease in the rate of contraction of rat cardiomyocytes and loss of synchronous beating (Williamson et al., 2001). Secondary bile acids, lithocholic acid (LCA) and deoxicholic acid (DCA) which are also elevated in patients with ICP, are able to cross the placenta (Heikkinen et al., 1980). These compounds have been shown to be fetotoxic in experimental animals causing embrio death, birth deformities and fetal growth restriction (Zimber et al., 1990).

In vitro studies indicate that myometrial cell preparations from ICP women show a more intense response to oxytocin stimuli than do cells from healthy women (Israel et al., 1986) and an increase of oxytocin-receptor expression after being incubated with CA (Germain et al., 2003). These findings could be related with preterm delivery in ICP although the exact mechanism of action is still unclear for a complete explanation.

2. Diagnosis and treatment

Usually, diagnosis of ICP is based on pruritus with mild or moderate elevated levels of amino transferases and raised total serum bile acids (TSBA) (Reyes et al., 1993). However, it is often difficult to accomplish an accurate diagnosis by performing solely routine laboratory tests because they are also altered in some other conditions of pregnancy. In fact, the existence of subclinical cholestasis during pregnancy may also make difficult the diagnosis of the disease. Moreover, pruritus in pregnancy is a common symptom in ICP but this evidence is not sufficient to discriminate women with ICP from those with benign condition of pruritus gravidarum (Meng et al., 1997, Castaño et al., 2006).

A number of other disorders may erroneously be interpreted as ICP during pregnancy: skin diseases, specific dermatoses of pregnancy, allergic reactions, renal pruritus and hematological disorders such as Hodkin´s disease and polycythemia rubra vera (Pusl et al., 2007). The most sensitive indicator in the diagnosis of ICP is a rise of serum bile acid levels. Total serum bile acids in healthy pregnancies are slightly higher in pregnant (6.6 ± 0.8 μM) than in non-pregnant women (3.2 ±0.7 μM) (Castaño et al., 2006) but levels up to 11.0 μM are accepted as normal in late gestation (Brites et al., 2002). Higher fetal complication rates have been associated with TSBA levels higher than 40 μM (Glanz et al., 2004, Pusl et al., 2007). Spontaneous preterm deliveries, asphyxia events and meconium staining of amniotic fluid, placenta and membranes increased by 1-2% for each additional μmol/L of total bile acid concentrations. However, these events did not increase until bile acid levels exceeded 40 μM (Glanz et al., 2004). It is suggested that patients could be expectantly managed when TSBA levels remain below 40 μM and when pregnant women refer pruritus it should be surveilled with the aid of repeated determinations of serum bile acids.(Glantz et al., 2004)

Recently, a subgroup of asymptomatic pregnant women with high levels of TSBA, and normal liver function tests but not showing pruritus has been classified as asymptomatic hypercholanaemic pregnants (AHP) (Castaño et al, 2006; Lunzer et al., 1986; Pascual et al., 2002; Tripodi et al., 2003). Women with AHP did not differ from normocholanemic women respect to clinical, biochemical or perinatal characteristics. AHP does not appear to be a clinical entity by itself, but a subgroup of normal pregnancies with higher levels of TSBA specially the conjugated dihydroxy serum bile acids (Castaño et al., 2006).

It has been reported that TSBA levels observed in ICP overlapped with those of healthy and AHP pregnant women, making it difficult to obtain a differential diagnosis on the basis of TSBA measurements as the key for recognition of the disease (Castaño et al., 2006, Muresan et al., 2007). Indeed, ICP may be present without elevated bile acids (Muresan et al., 2007; Egerman et al., 2004). It has also been reported that up to 45 % of patients with clinical diagnosis of ICP may have normal fasting serum bile acids (Mullaly et al., 2001).

Therefore a clear question emerges from these observations: the monitoring of the patient should be discontinued if the TSBA levels are within the reference values? What happen if these levels change over the course of the week of delivery?

With regard to this point, serum bile acid profile has proved to be more informative than the determination of TSBA (Baqc et al.; 1995, Meng et al., 1997; Castaño et al., 2006; Lucangioli et al., 2009). Although many authors agree on the benefits of evaluating serum bile acids individually, there is no consensus in assigning a particular bile acid determination as the most useful indication in order to diagnose ICP or in establishing adequate bile acids ratios to solve how to recognize the disease. One of the reasons of these differences could be attributed to different analytical methods reported with the purpose of evaluating the bile acid profiles or it could be due to ethnic differences that lead to different bile acid prevalences.

It is important to emphasize that the serum bile acid profile is useful not only to diagnose ICP but also to analyze the evolution of the disease after treatment (Castaño et al., 2006).

The pharmacological treatment of ICP with antihistamine, anion exchange resins and phenobarbital to remove peripheral pruritogens has not received wide acceptance because of their incomplete efficacy or side effects of therapy (Lammert et al., 2000). Cholestyramine is an anion exchange bile acid-binding resin giving some successful results in managing pruritus. However, this drug contributes to fat-soluble vitamin deficiency leading to postpartum hemorrhage, it does not correct liver enzyme abnormalities and it does not improve fetal prognosis in ICP (Mullally et al., 2001). Ursodeoxycholic acid (UDCA), a naturally hydrophilic bile acid is presently considered in the treatment of ICP because it improves clinical and biochemical parameters in pregnant women. The mechanisms of action of UDCA are still under discussion, but there are some evidences of protective and antioxioxidant effects of this bile acid (Lee et al., 1997; Brites, 2002; Copaci et al., 2005). It is also known that UDCA therapy alters the hydrophilicity and, therefore, the overall distribution of bile acids in the bile acid pool decreasing levels of hydrophobic and toxic bile acids as LCA (Lucangioli et al., 2009, Mullally et al., 2001). Moreover, it is known that UDCA reverse the impairment in the functionality of bile acid transport across the trophoblast, so its administration can be a valuable contribution to the fetal well-being (Serrano et al., 1998). On the other hand, UDCA has been shown to improve impaired hepatocellular secretion by mainly posttranscriptional stimulations of canalicular transporter proteins leading to enhance the elimination of bile acid metabolites and other organic anions as well as mono- and disulphate steroids (Pusl et al., 2007). UDCA seems to be well tolerated by pregnant women and no adverse effect in mothers or newborns has been observed.

3. Bile Acids: Chemical structure and functions

Bile acids (BA) are steroid compounds pertaining to hydroxyl-derivatives of 5β-cholan-24-oic acid. They have different physico-chemical properties according to the number, position and orientation of their hydroxylgroups, and by conjugation with glycine and taurine, glyco-and tauro-derivatives are produced to the liver (Lucangioli et al., 2001). Figure 1 presents the chemical structures of bile acids showing primary BA like cholic acid (CA) and chenodeoxycholic acid (CDCA) and secondary BA, deoxycholic acid (DCA), lithocholic acid (LCA) and ursodeoxycholic (UDCA) (Tripodi et al., 2003). Moreover, BA are acidic molecules with pka values of 1.5 for taurine derivatives, 4.5 for glycine derivatives and 6 for unconjugated BA.

The biological functions of BA are principally associated with lipid digestion and absorption, solubilization of cholesterol and bile formation (Roda et al., 1995). Under physiological conditions, serum BA concentrations are normally present at micromolar level in the peripheral circulation. However, in hepatobiliary and intestinal diseases, the hepatic synthesis and clearance of BA and their intestinal absorption are disturbed, enabling quantitative and qualitative changes in the pattern of serum BA (Burkard et al., 2005).

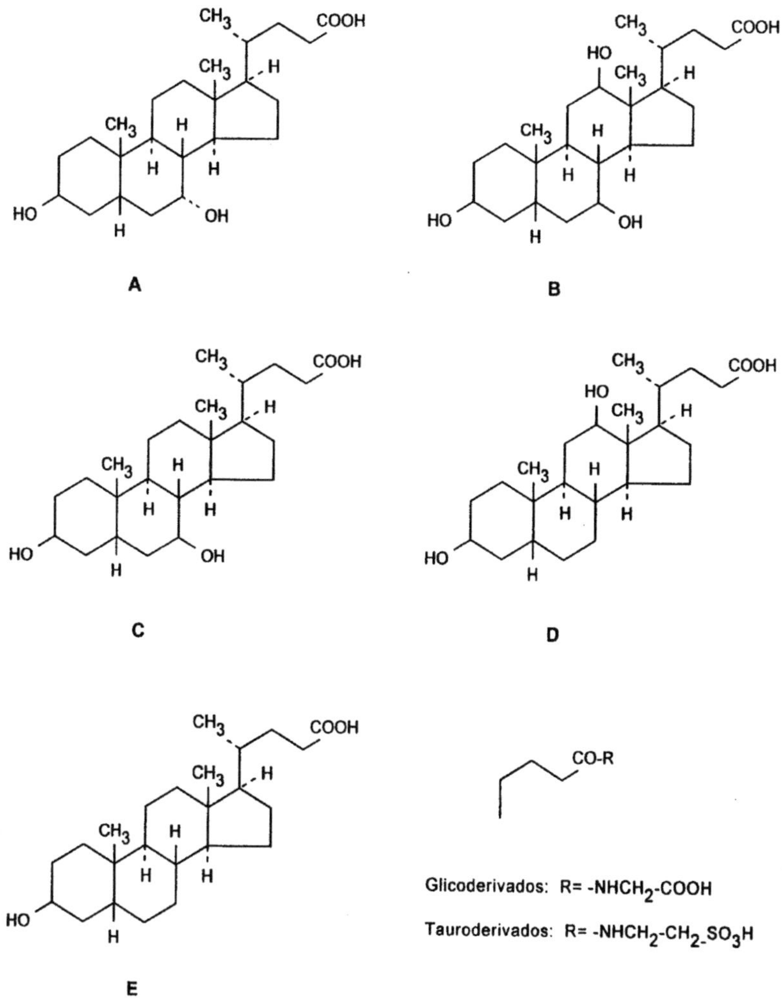

Fig. 1. Chemical structures of bile acids as free forms and their glyco-and tauroderivatives (A) UDCA, (B) CA, (C) CDCA, (D) DCA and (E) LCA

Regarding liver therapy, some BA, like UDCA and CDCA, are administered as therapeutic agents in the treatment of cholesterol gallstones. UDCA has also been used in the therapy of cholestatic liver disease (Konikoff, 2003; Paumgartner et al., 2004).

4. An overview of different analytical techniques in serum bile acid studies

4.1 Separative techniques

The analysis of BA is challenging since they are present at micromolar concentrations in biological fluids, and each BA has small structural differences between the others. Different analytical methods have been developed for the quantitation of BA in various matrices applying separative techniques. In this sense, high-performance liquid chromatography (HPLC) has been a popular technique applied in the individual analysis of BA in biological fluids. The HPLC- methods reported involve two chromatographic systems to determine the complete BA profile, one for free BA and the other system for BA derivatives (Vescina et al., 1993). Unfortunately, the combination of HPLC with UV-detection, limited the sensitivity of the analysis due to the fact that BA have little chromophorore groups in their molecules (Fig. 1). To improve sensitivity, some derivatization methods have been described by Burkard (Gatti et al., 1997). However, these methods are time consuming. In contrast, HPLC coupled to mass (MS) detector, represents a sensitive and selective chromatographic technique to determine BA in biological matrices. Several MS techniques by ionization have been used for BA analysis like HPLC-MS and HPLC-MS/MS, though specially applied to the analysis of BA derivatives (Bootsma et al., 1999; Tagliacozzi et al., 2003), being the electrospray ionization (ESI) the best detection system. In contrast, unconjugated BA are not detectable by MS/MS due to the lack of any specific fragment ions originated from their molecules. However, Burkard et al. have developed an HPLC-MS/MS method to quantify free and derivatives UDCA, CDCA and DCA in serum. Quantification of unconjugated BA was performed using single ion monitoring mode of the deprotonated molecules (Burkard et al., 2005).

Gas chromatography (GC), has also been applied to the analysis of BA in biological fluids (Batta et al., 1999), in some cases, coupling MS as detector (Niwa, 1995; Setchell,et al., 1983). However, GC-MS methods are not simple as they require an extensive sample pre-treatment like extraction, purification and hydrolysis of conjugated BA and the preparation of volatile derivatives prior to detection of all the products (Perwaiz et al., 2010).

Thin layer chromatography (TLC) is other separative technique applied to the quantitation of BA in biological matrix. This technique has used to determine conjugated and unconjugated BA, however, UDCA and CDCA cannot be resolved. Brites et al. applied TLC in combination with HPLC-UV and GC-MS to quantitate BA in different biological sample (Rodriguez et al., 1999). However, TLC is not widely extended in laboratories

4.1.1 Capillary electrophoresis

Capillary electrophoresis (CE) is a family of related techniques that employs narrow-bore capillaries to perform high efficiency separations of both large and small molecules, favoured by the use of high voltages, which may generate electroosmotic and electrophoretic flows of buffer solutions and ionic species, respectively, within the capillary.

The CE advantages with respect to other analytical techniques, such as very high resolution in short time of analysis, versatility, the possibility to analyze molecules without chromophore groups, simultaneous analysis of various compounds with different hydrophobic characteristics, small volume of sample, and low cost, have made this technique adequate for the analysis of numerous types of compounds like biological macromolecules, chiral compounds, inorganic ions, organic acids, DNA fragments and even whole cells and virus particles. An increasing number of applications of CE are in progress in many clinical laboratories. Significant potential benefits in the future will impact on clinical diagnosis and therapy. Specially, there are several instances in which the limited availability of biological fluids significantly preclude the analysis of various relevant biochemical compounds that can be achieved because small volumes of sample are required by this technique.

Over the last 20 years, capillary electrophoresis has evolved into a powerful analysis technique with different applications. Firstly created to be focused on water-soluble ionic analysis, CE has grown to a very high degree of development and now it is employed in a wide variety of pharmaceutical, biopharmaceutical and clinical applications. Its development in today´s world is in the step of miniaturization processes in science and technology including analytical chemistry.

Medical diagnosis and quality control assays are areas that are specially benefited from miniaturization. The ability to quantify each time smaller amounts of compounds in biological fluids together with the capacity of analytical systems to handle low nanoliter sample volumes extremely improve the diagnosis of many diseases.

The main disadvantage in the analysis of biological samples are the following: a) small amounts of biological fluids or tissues available, that usually are not enough to determine their components by traditional techniques; b) small quantities of these components that, in some cases, are present in trace amounts; c) presence of numerous interferences and d) requirement of simultaneous separation and determination of more than one component. These are the major reasons for calling this type of sample as a "complex matrix".

In clinical applications, the analytical system should be capable of handling nanoliter volumes of sample, effective enough to determine analytes at subnanomolar concentrations, and should provide high selectivity and successful separations of different molecules in a single run.

Capillary electrophoresis seems to possess many of the advantages required for a nanotechnique employed with clinical purpose.

A CE system has been developed for the analysis of BA profile in plasma. The CE system is based on a micellar electrokinetic chromatography, as a mode of CE, with the use of sodium dodecyl sulfate as micellar agent and cyclodextrins (CD-MEKC) (Tripodi et al., 2003) using UV detection. The CD-MEKC system allowed the simultaneous and complete resolution of 15 BA (taurine, glycine and unconjugted BA) in serum sample in less than 12 min with good precision and accuracy using a simple sample preparation (Fig. 2).

4.2 Enzymatic assay

Enzymatic methods have been used to determine total BA in biological matrices. A NAD-dependent steroid dehydrogenase, oxidizes hydroxycholanoates with formation of NADH, which is measured by UV or fluorimetric methods (Griffiths et al., 2010). 3∞-hydroxysteroid dedydrogenase is used in clinical chemistry for analysis of plasma BA to monitor changes in liver diseases, however, only BA with 3∞- hydroxysteroid in its molecule can be determined.

4.3 Immunoassays

Many radioimmunoassay and enzyme immunoassays methods have been applied for simple and rapid analysis of common total BA in plasma. An important disadvantage of these methods is specificity, particularly at low concentrations of BA (Griffiths et al., 2010).

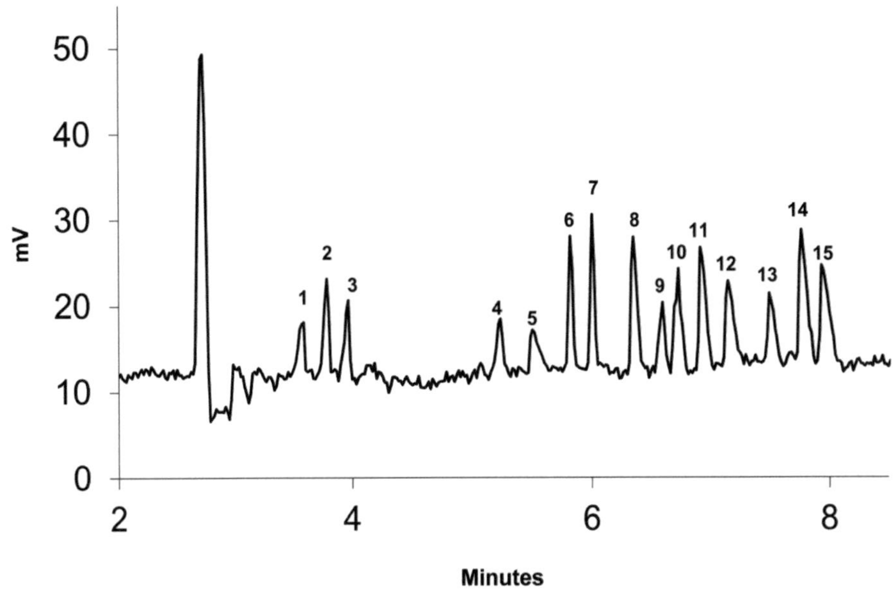

A): Electropherogram of a serum sample matrix spiked with 15 bile acid standards, 6-10µM for free bile acids and 4-6µM for conjugated bile acids. 1: UDCA, 2: GUDCA, 3: TUDCA, 4: LCA, 5: CDCA, 6: GLCA, 7: TLCA, 8: GCDCA, 9: CA, 10: TCDCA, 11: DCA, 12: GCA, 13: TCA, 14: GDCA, 15: TDCA

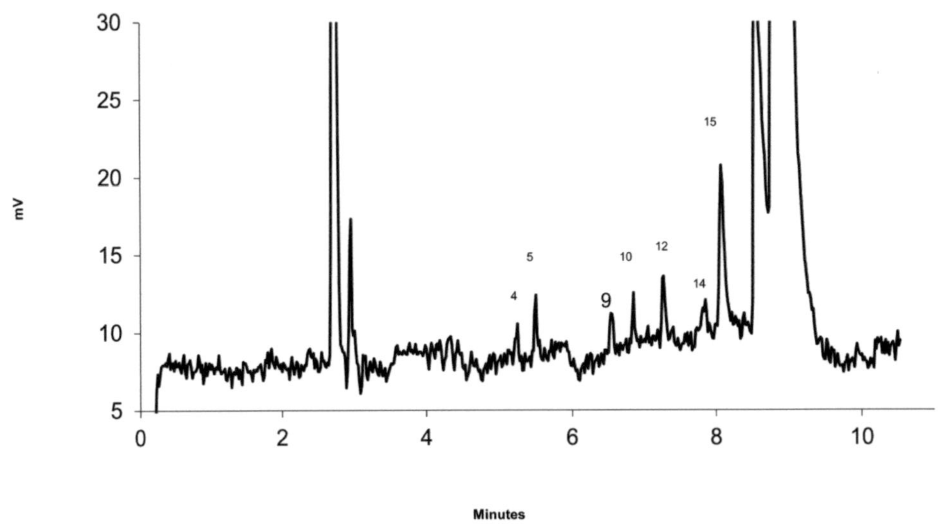

B): Electropherogram of a serum sample from an ICP patient. 4: LCA, 5: GLCA, 9: CA, 10: TCDCA, 12: GCA, 14: GDCA, 15: TDCA

Fig. 2. Electropherograms of serum bile acid assessed by capillary electrophoresis

5. Clinical interpretation of serum bile acid profile

Although physicians have so far used TSBA levels in the diagnosis of ICP, there is sufficient evidence that they are not efficient enough as it would be expected. A single value of TSBA could be replaced by assessing the profile of bile acids or certain ratios calculated between certain BA in particular. It is therefore a priority for physicians to take into account these results and interpret correctly the laboratory data for a better evaluation and control of the ICP disease. However, not all researchers agree on which bile acid provides more information, possibly because of methodological differences in addition to ethnic characteristics that might have influence on serum bile acid profiles from different populations of the world.

Laatikaimen et al. in 1978 and many other authors later (Laatikaimen et al., 1978, Brites et al., 1998, Bacq et al., 1995) showed a marked predominance of CA in ICP while Castaño et al (2006) demonstrated the presence of LCA as the preponderant bile acid in this disorder. Brites et al. in 1998 showed that elevations of glycocholic acid provide a sensitive biochemical test for the diagnosis of ICP with 95 % efficiency but state that TCA is even better having 100% efficiency (Brites et al., 1998). There are several reports which have demonstrated that different ratios calculated from individual bile acid determinations are useful in the comprehension of different types of liver diseases (Brites et al., 1998, Azer et al., 1997, Pusl et al., 2007). Heikkinen in 1983 and later Brites in 1998 (Heikkinen, 1983; Brites et al., 1998) demonstrated that the CA/CDCA ratio is increased in ICP approximately from 4:1 to 8:1 respect to normal pregnancies.

Brites et al (1998) employed HPLC for conjugated bile acids analysis and TLC for free bile acids, highlighting that free UDCA was not quantified because it did not separate from CDCA during TLC separation. On the basis of this methodology the authors established that better criterium to diagnose ICP is TSBA >11μM, CA/CDCA >1.5, %CA>42%, Glycine/Taurine <1 and GCA/TCA>2.

However, a latter report has recently determined that CA / CDCA ratio contribute little to the diagnosis of ICP (Huang et al., 2009). Using capillary electrophoresis as analytical technique, it has been demonstrated not only that CA/ CDCA ratio was below the unit but also a shift towards a hydrophobic composition with higher levels of LCA and free bile acids was found in women with ICP concluding that LCA is a useful parameter in the differential diagnosis of ICP and AHP (Castaño et al., 2006).

With regard to the analysis of serum bile acids it was found that AHP women showed TSBA levels above the usually accepted cut-off values and their serum bile acid profiles demonstrated that UDCA levels were higher in AHP patients compared to normal pregnant women and to all ICP patients before treatment, with either low or high score pruritus (table 1). Moreover, in AHP patients LCA levels showed no difference with values of normal pregnant women (Castaño et al., 2006). An inspection of the UDCA /LCA ratio, the highest value was observed in AHP patients because of the increment of UDCA levels observed in these patients. It could be possible to hypothesize that this high ratio has a protective effect in AHP patients since they do not develop ICP even with elevated TSBA and it is possible that UDCA/LCA ratio could have a higher discrimination power than individual bile acid determinations. These evidences should be demonstrated in further studies.

	Non-pregnant women (n=10)	Normocholamenic (n=18)	AHP (n=12)	ICP (n=41)
Total SBA (μM)	3.2 ± 0.7	6.6 ± 0.8	21.9 ± 3.2	29.5 ± 3.3
LCA (μM)	0.05 ± 0.06	0.3 ± 0.2	0.10 ± 0.03	8.2 ± 1.7
CDCA (μM)	0.9 ± 0.4	0.7 ± 0.3	3.3 ± 2.1	4.2 ± 0.9
DCA (μM)	0.2 ± 0.1	1.3 ± 0.7	4.0 ± 1.2	4.9 ± 1.1
CA (μM)	0.7 ± 0.4	0.7 ± 0.1	1.1 ± 0.7	3.6 ± 0.8
UDCA (μM)	0.9 ± 0.3	4.5 ± 0.9	13.3 ± 1.9	8.5 ± 1.6
Free/conjugated	1.1 ± 0.3	0.05 ± 0.02	0.3 ± 0.1	1.3 ± 0.3
Taurine/Glycine	5.0 ± 0.2	5.6 ± 0.2	6.7 ± 0.2	5.7 ± 0.1

Table 1. Comparison of TSBA levels and SBA profiles in different groups studied. Results are expressed as means ± SEM. Bile acids are expressed in their free, glycine and taurine forms. From reference Castaño 2006.

Later, the same authors (Lucangioli et al., 2009) proposed LCA as an alternative biomarker and a more sensitive parameter to evaluate effectiveness of UDCA treatment. It was observed a relief of pruritus together with a dramatic decrease in LCA concentrations in all patients following UDCA therapy (Fig 3). It was also found that TSBA concentrations overlapped before and after UDCA therapy (Fig. 4). Instead, LCA concentrations were high in all ICP patients but decreased only in the group of treated patients. Thus, the mentioned results indicated that LCA is a more sensitive marker than TSBA to evaluate the therapeutic monitoring of ICP. In the same work the authors observed that a decrease in the

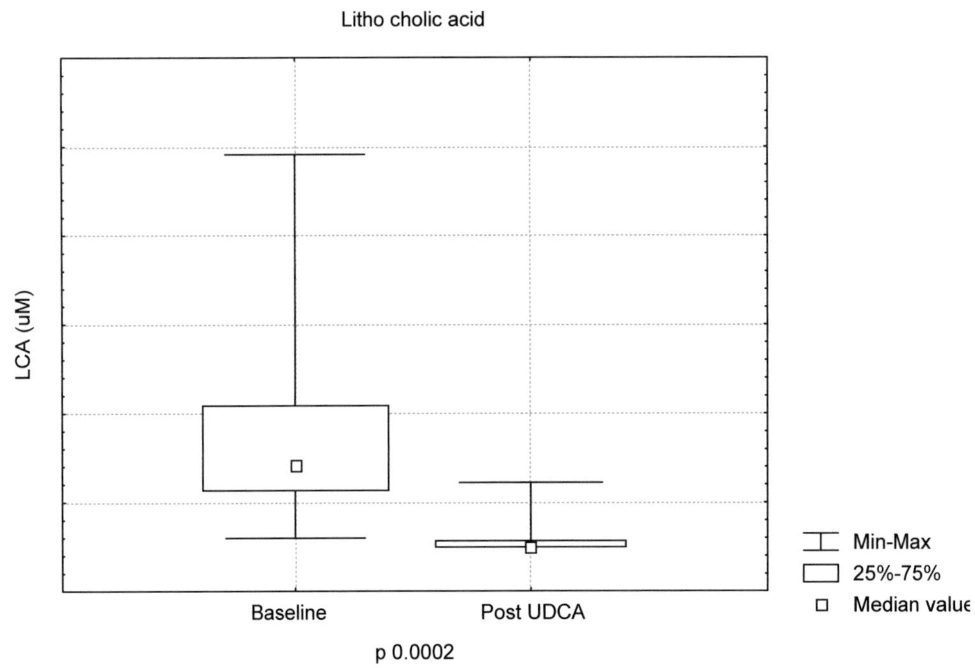

Fig. 3. The effect of UDCA therapy in LCA

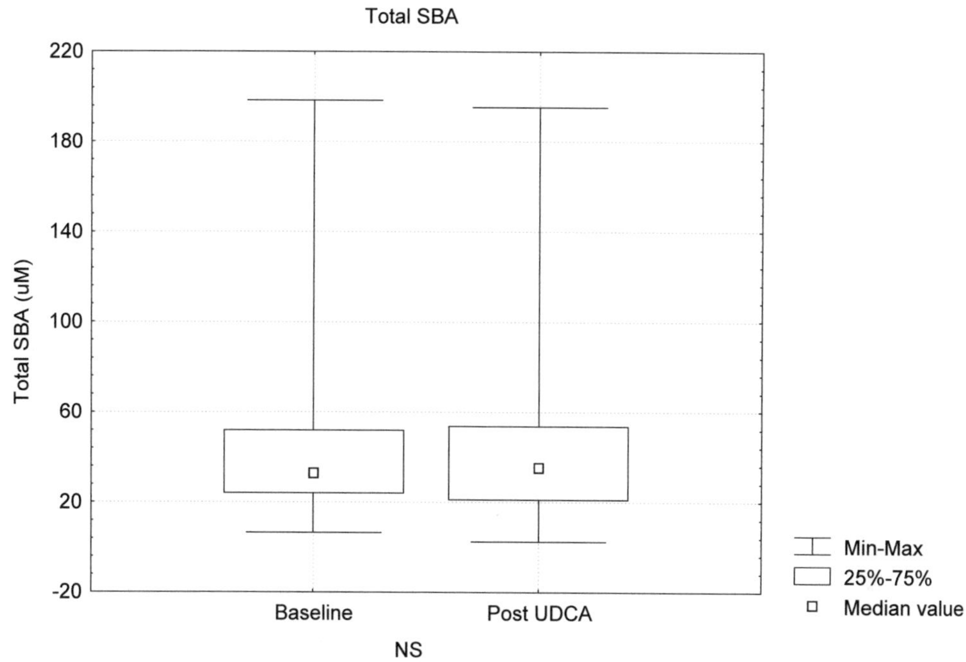

Fig. 4. The effect of UDCA therapy in TSBA

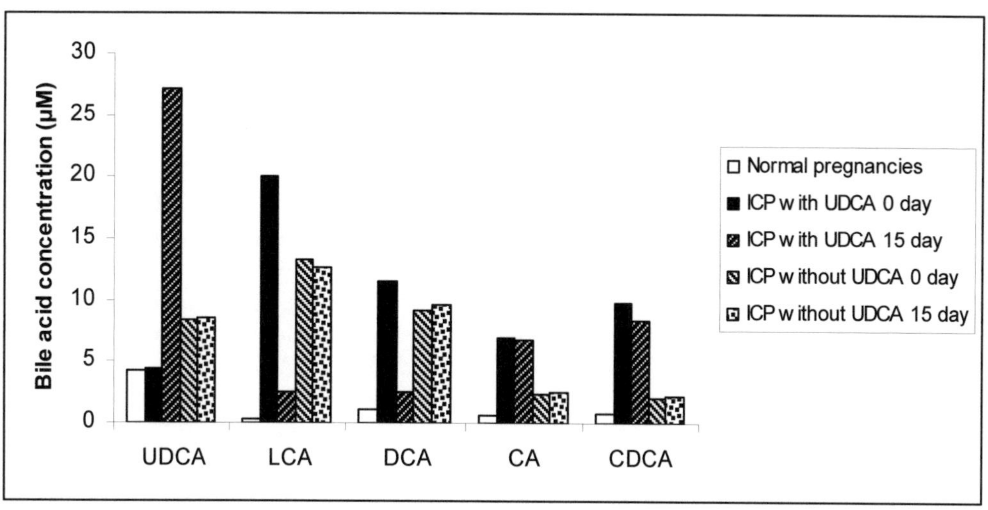

Fig. 5. Comparison of SBA profiles (mean ± SEM) in normal pregnancies (n = 20) and ICP patients with (n =23) and without (n = 5) UDCA treatment. Bile acids are expressed as the sum of their free, glycine and taurine forms. *p<0.001 (difference in LCA from day 0 to 15 with UDCA treatment), **p<0.03 (difference in DCA from day 0 to 15 with UDCA treatment)

concentrations obtained in individual SBA did not have any time effect, since SBA profiles in ICP patients without therapy did not change during 15 days (Fig 5). This result showed that the decrease in LCA and DCA concentrations could be attributed only to UDCA treatment (Lucangioli et al, 2009).

In conclusion, although there is no consensus about which bile acids are better indicators for evaluating the ICP, it must be emphasized that clinicians should gradually abandon using the value of TSBA determination to assess bile acid profile as a more accurate approach in ICP diagnosis and treatment.

6. References

Altshuler G and Hyde S. (1989) Meconium-induced vasocontraction: a potential cause of cerebral and other fetal hypoperfusion and of poor pregnancy outcome. J. Child Neurol. 4, 137-142.

Altshuler G, Arizawa M. and Molnar-Nadasdy G. (1992) Meconium-induced umbilical cord cascular necrosis and ulceration: a potential link between the placenta and poor pregnancy outcome. Obstet. Gynecol. 79, 760-766.

Azer S., Klaassen C. and Stacey N. (1997) biochemical assay of serum bile acids: methods and applications. Br. J. Biomed Sci. 54, 118-132.

Bacq, Y., Myara, A., Brechot, M., Hamon, C., Studer, E. Trivin, F. and Metman E. (1995) Serum conjugated bile acid profile during intrahepatic cholestasis of pregnancy. J. of Hepatol. 22, 66-70.

Batta A. and Salen G. (1999) Gas chromatography of bile acids. J Chromatogr. B Biomed Sci Appl. 723, 1-16.

Bootsma A., Overmars H, van Rooij A, van Lint A., Wanders R., van Gennip A., Vreken P. (1999) Rapid analysis of conjugated bile acids in plasma using electrospray tandem mass spectrometry: application for selective screening of peroxisomal disorders. J. Inherit, Metab Dis. 22, 307-10.

Brites D. (2002) Intrahepatic cholestasis of pregnancy: changes in materal-fetal bile acid balance and improvement by ursodeoxycholic acid. Ann. Hepatol. 1(1), 20-28.

Brites D., Rodrigues C., Oliveira N., Cardoso M. and Graça (1998) Correction of maternal serum bile acid profile during ursodeoxycholic acid therapy in cholestasis of pregnancy. J. Hepatol. 28, 91-98.

Brites D., Rodrigues C., van-Zeller H., Briyo A. and Silva R. (1998) Relevance of serum bile acid profile in the diagnosis of intrahepatic cholestasis of pregnancy in an high incidence area: Portugal. Obstet. Gynecol. 80, 31-38.

Brites, D., Rodriguez, C., Cardoso, M and Graca, L. (1998). Unusual case of severe cholestasis of pregnancy with early onset improved by ursodeoxycholic acid administration. Eir. J. Obstet. Gynecol. Reprod. Biol. 72, 165-168.

Burkard I., von Eckardstein A. and Rentsch K. (2005) Differentiated quantification of human bile acids in serum by high-performance liquid chromatography-tandem mass spectrometry. J. Chromatogr. B. 826, 147-159.

Castaño G., Lucangioli S., Sookoian S, Mesquida M., Lemberg A., Di Scala M., Franchi P., Carducci C. And Tripodi V. (2006) Bile acid profiles by capillary electrophoresis in intrahepatic cholestasis of pregnancy. Clin Sci. 110, 459-465.

Copaci I, Lauentjiu M, Iliescu L and Voiculescu M. (2005) New therapeutical indications of ursodeoxycholic acid. J. Gastroenterol. 14 (3), 259-266.

Diaferia, A., Nicastri, P., Tartagni, M., Loizzi, P., Iacovizzi, C.and Di Leo, A. (1996) Ursodeoxycholic acid therapy in pregnant women with cholestasis. Int. J. of Gynecol and Obstet. 52, 133-140.

Egerman R. and Reily C. (2004) Predicting fetal outcome in intrahepatic cholestasis of pregnancy: Is the bile acid level sufficient? Hepatology 40, 287-288.

Gatti, R, Toda A., Cerre D., Bonazzi D. and Cavrini V. (1997) HPLC-fluorescence determination of individual free and conjugated bile acids in human serum.Biomed Chromatogr. 11, 11-15.

Germain A, Kato S., Carvajal J., Valenzuela G., Valdes, G. And Glasinovic J. (2003) Am. J. Obstet. Gynecol., 189, 577-582.

Glantz A., Marschall H. and Mattsson L. (2004) Intrahepatic cholestasis of pregnancy: relationships between bile acid levels and fetal complication rates. Hepatology 40 (2). 467-474.

Griffiths W. and Sjövall J. (2010) Bile acids: analysis in biological fluids and tissues. J. Lipid Res. 51 (1), 23-41.

Heikkinen J. (1983) Serum bile acids in the early diagnosis of intrahepatic cholestasis of pregnancy. Obstet. Gynecol. 61. 581-587.

Heikkinen J., Maentausta O., Tuimala R., Ylöstalo P. and Jänne O. (1980) Amniotic fluid bile acids in normal and pathologic pregnancy. Obstet. Gynecol. 56, 60-84.

Huang W., Gowda M, Donnelly J. Bile acid ratio in diagnosis of intrahepatic cholestasis of pregnancy. Am. J. Perinatol. 26(4), 291-4.

Israel E., Guzman M. and Campos G (1986) Maximal response to oxytocine of the isolated myometrium from pregnant patients with intrahepatic cholestasis. Acta Obstet Gynecol. Scand. 65, 581-582

Konikoff F. (2003) Gallstones - approach to medical management. MedGenMed. 15;5(4):8.

Laatikainen T., Peltonen J. and Nylander P. (1974) Effect of maternal intrahepatic cholestasis on fetal steroid metabolism. J. Clin. Invest. 53, 1709-1715.

Laatikanen T., Lehtonen P. and Hesso A. (1978) Biliary bile acids in uncomplicated pregnancy and in cholestasis of pregnancy. Clin. Chem. Acta 85, 145-150

Lammert F., Marschall H., Glantz A. and Matern S. (2000) Intrahepatic cholestasis of pregnancy: molecular pathogenesis, diagnosis and management. J. of Hepatol. 33, 1012-1021.

Lee B., New A. and Ong C (1997) Comparative analysis of conjugated bile acids in human serum using high-performance liquid chromatography and capillary electrophoresis. J Chromatogr. B Biomed. Sci. Appl. 704, 35-42.

Lucangioli S., Castaño G., Contin M. and Tripodi V. (2009) Lithocholic acid as a biomarker of intrahepatic cholestasis of pregnancy during ursodeoxycholic acid treatment. Ann. Clin. Biochem. 46, 44-49.

Lucangioli, S., Carducci, C., Tripodi, V. and Kenndler E. (2001) Retention of bile salts in micellar electrokinetic chromatography: relation of capacity factor to octanol-water partition coefficient and critical concentration. J. Chromatogr. B, 765, 113-120.

Lunzer M., Barnes P., Byth K. and O'Halloran M. (1986) Serum bile acid concentrations during pregnancy and their relationship to obstetric cholestasis. Gastroenterology 91, 825-829.

Lutz E. and Margolis A. (1969) Obstetric hepatosis: treatment with cholestiramine and interim response to steroids. Obstet. Gynecol. 33, 64-71.

Meng, L., Reyes, H and Palma, J. (1997) Effects of ursodeoxycholic acid on conjugated bile acids and progesterone metabolites in serum and urine of patients with intrahepatic cholestasis of pregnancy. J. of Hepatol. 27, 1029-1040.

Milkiewicz, P., Elias, E., Williamson, C. and Weaver, J. (2002) Obstetric cholestasis. May have a sedious consequences for the fetus, and needs to be taken seriously.BMJ 324, 123-124

Mullally B., Hansen W. (2001) Intrahepatic cholestasis of pregnancy: review of the literature. Obstet and Gynecol. Survey 57 (1), 47-52.

Muresan D., Ona D, Cruciat G, Rotar I. And Stamatian F. (2007) Recurrent Intrahepatic cholestasis of pregnancy. A case report. J. Gastrointetin liver Dis. 17 (3), 323-325.

Niwa T. (1995) Procedures for MS analysis of clinically relevant compounds. Clin. Chim Acta 240, 75-152.

Pascual M., Serrano M., El-Mir, M., Macias R., Jimenez F. And Marin J. (2002) Relationship between asymptomatic hypercholanaenia of pregnancy and progesterone metabolism. Clin. Sci. 102, 587-593.

Paumgartner G. and Beuers U. (2004) Mechanisms of action and therapeutic efficacy of ursodeoxycholic acid in cholestatic liver disease.Clin. Liver Dis. 8, 67-81

Perwaiz S., Tuchweber B, Mignault D., Gilat T. and Yousef I. (2001) Determination of bile acids in biological fluids by liquid chromatography-electrospray tandem mass spectrometry. J. Lipid Res. 42, 114-119.

Pradhan, P. (2002). Obstetric cholestasis. J. of Nepal Med. Association 41, 335-340.

Pusl T and Beuers U. (2007) Intrahepatic cholestasis of pregnancy. Orphanet J. of Rare Dis. 2, 26-31.

Reyes H. and Simon F. (1993) Intrahepatic cholestasis of pregnancy: an estrogen-related disease. Semin. Liver Dis. 13, 289-301.

Roda A., Gioacchini A., Manetta A., Cerre C., Montagnani M. and Fini A. (1995) Bile acids: physico-chemical properties, function and activity. Ital. J. Gastroenterol. 27, 327-331

Rodriguez C., Marin J., Brites D. (1999) Bile acid patterns in meconium are influenced by cholestasis of pregnacy and not altered by ursodeoxycholic acid treatment. Gut 45, 446-452.

Serrano M., Brites D., Larena M Monte M., Bravo M. Oliveira N. and Marin J. (1998) Beneficial effect of ursodeoxychilic acid on alterations induced by cholestasis of pregnancy in bile acid transport across the human placenta. J Hepatol. 28, 829-839.

Serrano M., Brites D., Larena M., Monte M., Bravo M., Oliveira N. and Marin J. (1998) Effect of ursodeoxycholic acid treatment during intrahepatic cholestasis of pregnancy on the kinetics of bile acid transport across the placenta. J. Hepatol. 28 (5), 829-839.

Setchell K. and Matsui A. (1983) Serum bile acid analysis. Clin. Chim Acta 127, 1-17.

Shaw, D., Frohlich, J., Wittmann, B. and Williams, M. (1982). A prospective study of 18 patients with cholestasis of pregnancy. Am. J. Obstet. Gynecol. 142, 621-625.

Sjövall J. and Sjövall K. (1970) Steroid sulphates in plasma from pregnant women with pruritus and elevated plasma bile acid levels. Clin. Res. 2, 321-337-

Tagliacozzi D., Mozzi A., Casetta B., Bertucci P., Bernardini S. Di Ilio C, Urbani A. and Federici G. (2003) Quantitative analysis of bile acids in human plasma by liquid chromatography-electrospray tandem mass spectrometry: a simple and rapid one-step method. Clin. Chem Lab. Med. 41, 1633-41

Tripodi V., Lucangioli S., Scioscia S. and Carducci C. (2003) Simultaneous determination of free and conjugated bile acids in serum by cyclodextri-modified micellar electrokinetic chromatography. J. Chromatography B, 785, 147-155.

Vescina M., Mamianetti A., Vizioli N., Lucangioli S., Rodriguez V., Orden A., Garrido D. and Carducci C. (1993) Evaluation of faecal bile acid profiles by HPLC after using disposable solid-phase columns. Journal of Pharmaceutical and Biomedical Analysis, 11 (11/12), 1331-1335.

Williamson C., Gorelik J, Eaton B., Lab M. Swiet M. and Korchev Y. (2001) The bile acid taurocholate impairs rat cardiomyocyte function: a proposed mechanism for intra-uterine fetal death in obstetric cholestasis. Clin Sci. 100, 363-369.

Zimber A. and Zusman I (1990) Effect of secondary bile acids on the intrauterine development in rats. Teratology, 42, 215-224.

2

Iatrogenic Bile Duct Injuries Following Laparoscopic Cholecystectomy: Myth or Reality? A Recent Literature Review from 2006 to 2011

Giovanni Conzo, Salvatore Napolitano, Giancarlo Candela, Antonietta Palazzo, Francesco Stanzione, Claudio Mauriello and Luigi Santini
7th Division of General Surgery, School of Medicine
Second University of Naples, Naples
Italy

1. Introduction

At the end of 1980's, the introduction of mininvasive surgery in clinical practice represented a significant achievement of science and technology research, and laparoscopic cholecystectomy (LC) is nowadays considered a gold standard in the treatment of symptomatic cholelithiasis, according to well known and acknowledged advantages. Although experience is essential to avoiding rates of morbidity in any surgical procedure, in LC the effect of the learning curve does not seem to be the most important factor in minimizing the possibility of iatrogenic bile duct injuries (IBDI) because most of them are related to anatomic misdiagnoses and lapses from basic principles of biliary surgery. IBDI are still a severe complication of biliary surgery, characterized by high morbidity and in some cases significant mortality, often due to the onset of septic complications. They cause a costs rise, related to diagnostic and therapeutic procedures, and they are often associated with distressing litigations, frustrating for surgeons. Factors that may be related to IBDI include certain pitfalls believed to be inherent in the laparoscopic approach: the two-dimensional view and the absence of tactile sensation. However, an analysis of literature until 2005 shows that the "mini-invasive" approach is related to a higher incidence of iatrogenic bile duct injuries (IBDI), both of the main and accessory bile ducts. In 2002 Nuzzo (Nuzzo, 2002), by the means of an Italian survey, proved a three times higher incidence of IBDI than in open cholecystectomy (OC), showing about 300 bile duct injuries out of every 100000 cholecystectomies per year in Italy, pointing out in that country a considerable mortality, in most of cases related to sepsis, with a significant rise of morbidity and healthcare costs ensuing from hospital stay, instrumental investigations, and medium and long-term clinical follow-up. Moreover, IBDI are reported to have late severe aftermath, causing the surgeon frustration and expensive litigation. After accomplishing a learning curve for mini-invasive approach, led by an experienced surgeon, the most significant etiopathogenetic factors of IBDI are the misidentification of the main biliary tree (BT) and wrong manoeuvres to manage bleedings. Treatment of IBDI requires a multidisciplinary approach - namely endoscopy, interventional radiology and surgery - in referral centres, because in most cases the proper repair represents often the ultimate intervention to the patient. Whenever a surgical treatment is required - for "major" injuries - hepaticojejunostomy represents the best choice, but options are described as T-tube drainage, liver resections and even liver transplantation, confirming their potential extreme seriousness. Patients undergoing reparative interventions, following IBDI, require frequently a cholestasis evaluation by long-term clinical, biochemical and imaging follow-up (> 10 years), because of the possible onset of long term complications (anastomotic strictures, secondary biliary cirrhosis), that produce a significant growth of expenditures. Authors performed a meta-analysis of most recent reviews articles of the last five years, with the aim of assessing the real incidence of this issue during these late years.

2. Methods

A Pubmed database search was performed to identify the most recent articles from 2006 to 2011, about IBDI following cholecystectomy, using the keywords "laparoscopic cholecystectomy", "small-incision cholecystectomy", "open cholecystectomy", "iatrogenic bile duct injuries", "biliary fistulas", "iatrogenic biliary strictures", and "cholestasis". Additional papers, among the most important and cited in literature, reporting incidence of BDI following LCs, were individually searched for, excluding case report articles. These data are purely descriptive and no statistical analysis was performed. We excluded "Single-Port cholecystectomy" from our research. By the means of this research, authors examined the incidence, the main risk factors, the mechanisms of bile duct injuries, the diagnostic work-up and the management, in order to provide the most recent results about this issue.

3. Classification of IBDI

At present several classifications of IBDI have been proposed with the aim of standardizing the assessment, planning treatment and evaluating the outcome. Nevertheless, none of these have been universally accepted as a standard. Some of these classifications are based on the anatomical level of the lesion (Strasberg et al., 1995), (Bismuth, 1982), (Neuhaus et al., 2000), (Csendes et al., 2001), (McMahon et al., 1995), (Siewert et al., 1994), (Frattaroli et al., 1996) and (Bergman et al., 1996) and on the kind of repair required. On the other hand, other classifications - (Bektas et al., 2007), (Lau & Lei, 2007), (Kapoor, 2008),(Stewart-Way, 2004) - also assess hilar vascular lesions associated in IBDI, which could jeopardize their management and overall morbidity. None of them include factors such as sepsis, haemodynamic status or comorbidities, which affect remarkably long-term outcome. The most commonly used is Strasberg classification (1995), which incorporates the previous classification of Bismuth (1982). The development of these two classifications kept up with the operative technique, because thanks to LC, IBDI became more complex and more proximal than in OC, so requiring an assessment both of site and type of lesion, from the transection through wrong closures, up to strictures. The authors prefer Strasberg classification not only for its feasibility to figure out the proper treatment, but also because most vascular injuries occurring in LC don't modify the repair technique of the biliary tree. Type A injuries include cystic duct leakage or leakage from canalicula in the liver bed, and these can be treated by endoscopy (papillotomy and prosthesis). Type B consists of partial occlusion of the biliary tree, mainly caused by the closure of an aberrant right hepatic duct. Type C includes the transection without ligation of the aberrant right hepatic duct. Type D describes partial damages to a major hepatic duct. Types E injuries are further subdivided into E1 through E5 according to the previous Bismuth classification: E1, transection of bile duct > 2 cm from the hilum; E2, transection of bile duct < 2 cm from the hilum; E3 and E4 represent stricture at the same level or above the confluence of hepatic ducts; E5 injuries describe involvement of an aberrant right sectoral duct injury concomitant with a common hepatic duct stricture.

Author	Year	Incidence	Operations
Giger	2006	0,3	22953
Koulas	2006	0,1	925
Plummer	2006	0,02	350
Nickkholgh	2006	0,09	2130
Tan	2006	0,5	202
Ledniczky	2006	0,1	1002
Hussain	2006	0,4	725
Yüksel	2006	0	74
Wenner	2006	0	338
Sarli	2006	0,16	2538
Velanovic	2006	0,25	3285
Hobbs	2006	0,26	19414
Santibane	2006	0,14	6107
Boddy	2007	0,4	4139
Karvonen	2007	0,38	3736
Lien	2007	0,12	5200
Cai	2007	0	629
Marakis	2007	0,16	1225
Yegiyants	2008	0,03	3042
Ibrahim	2008	0,4	1000
Malik	2008	1,67	1132
Yaghoubian	2008	0,7	2470
Georgiad	2008	0,69	2184
Veen	2008	1	1254
Tantia	2008	0,39	13305
Avgerinos	2009	0	1046
Machi	2009	0	1381
Triantafylli	2009	0,1	1009
Priego	2009	0,3	3933
Sanjay	2010	0	447
Yamashita	2010	0,58	n.d
Zha	2010	0,085	13000
Al-Kubati	2010	0,4	336
Ghnnam	2010	0,6	340
Gurusamy	2010	0,95	451
Keus	2010	0,7	2139
Giger	2011	0,3	31838
Pfluke	2011	0	65
Hamad	2011	0,18	2714
Harrison	2011	0,25	234220
Harboe	2011	0,2	20307
Stanisić	2011	0,2	386

Table 1. Incidence of IBDI reported in the literature from 2006 to 2011. Median incidence: 0,2% - Total amount of patients: 412585.

4. Analysis of IBDI incidence

Since its introduction over 20 years ago, population-based studies have reported a significant increase of IBDI incidence following LC, compared to open technique, ranging from 0,1% to 1,7%. About this issue, in Italy Nuzzo (Nuzzo et al., 2002) reported a three times higher incidence (0,3% vs 0,1%) compared to the conventional approach. Consequently, IBDI during LCs became an important issue in the field of surgical pathology. Although there was no evidence of superiority over open technique, soon after its introduction LC became the standard treatment of cholecystectomy (NIH Consensus Conference 1993). The rising popularity was based on assumed lower morbidity and complication proportions, and a quicker postoperative recovery compared to open technique (Sheha, 1996). However, the reviewed studies were non-randomised trials, with no fair assessment of the effects of the interventions. Authors carried out a survey of studies published from 2006 to 2011 (Table 1) (Figure 1), showing in the several surgical experiences an higher incidence during the early stage of learning, a following period of stabilisation, and an eventual decrease when the amount of LCs rose (Figure 2). In disagreement with this point of view, Giger (Giger, 2011) in a retrospective ten years survey (from 1995 to 2005) did not report a decrease of IBDI rates (0,3%), in spite of the assistance of the intraoperative cholangiography (IOC), considered useful for preventing iatrogenic injuries. However,

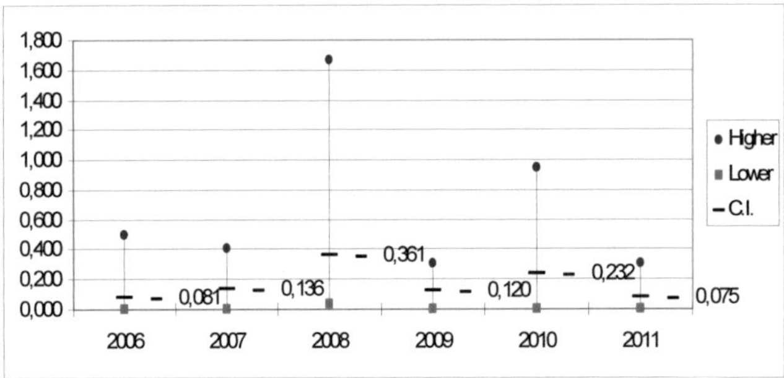

Fig. 1. IBDI incidence: analysis of literature from 2006 to 2011 C.I.: Confidence Interval 95%

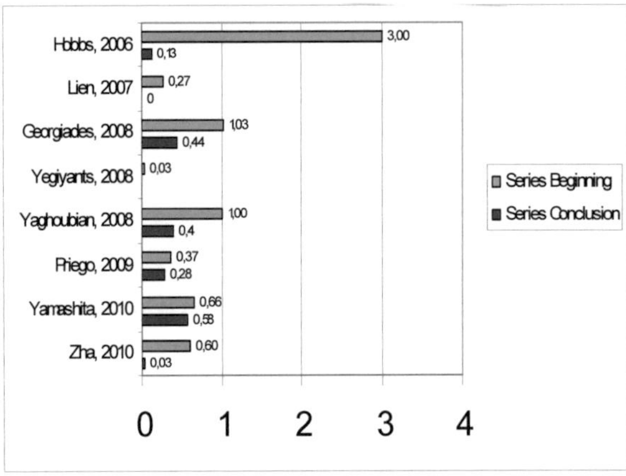

Fig. 2. IBDI incidence: relationship with surgical experience

several studies (with no statistical evidence) hypothesize that the regular practice of critical view of safety (CVS)- a codified dissective technique showing the anatomic elements of Calot's triangle- could cause a decrease of IBDI rates (Yamashita 2010, Yegiyants 2008, Avgerinos 2009, Sanjay 2010). Instead, Strasberg himself mentioned the lack of evidence of CVS for preventing IBDI, although surely a great step toward a safer LC, but it is unclear whether the CVS alone is sufficient as a technique to minimize the risk of IBDI. Also, by way of example, major IBDI continue to occur in the Netherlands despite increasing adoption of the CVS technique (de Reuver, 2007). Gurusamy (Gurusamy, 2010), in a meta-analysis of randomized clinical trials of LCs for acute cholecystitis, reports lower IBDI rates in early treted patients (0,5%) compared to delayed interventions (1,4%). Minor IBDI rates are also decreased according to Yüksel (Yüksel, 2006) (3% vs 4,6%). Boddy (Boddy, 2007) in a ten year series of 4139 LCs, reported lower rates of IBDI for hepatopancreaticobiliary surgeons (0,1%) in comparison to general surgery consultants (0,9%). Another controversial factor is the use of IOC: some authors recommend its routinary employment (Nickkholgh, 2006 - BDI 0,09%), others (Sarli, 2006) report no disadvantages with a selective use (IBDI 0,16%). About the influence of workload on surgeons efficiency, Yaghoubian (Yaghoubian, 2008) reports a decrease from 1% to 0,4% of IBDI, after implementation of the 80-hour workweek in his hospital. Two studies examine surgeon's experience as factor affecting IBDI incidence: Hobbs (Hobbs, 2006) reports a decrease of IBDI from 1994 to 1998 (from 0,35% to 0,13%), ascribing 1/3 of IBDI of his centre to surgeons with < 200 operations in the previous 5 years ; Harrison (Harrison, 2011), after analysing a 234280 LCs series, does not report any difference (IBDI 0,24% vs 0,26%) between rates of experienced surgeons compared to residents. Concerning the surgical approach, Keus' (Keus, 2010) Cochrane Review compares open, small-incision, and laparoscopic cholecystectomies, evaluating only randomized trials. In this study there is no statistical evidence of IBDI rates among the three approaches, with laparoscopic IBDI rates that range from 0,2% to 1,4%. However, the trials analysed in the review, statistically compelling, do not include acute cholecystitis as indication, but embrace minor injuries in IBDI rates, as self-limiting bile leakage, whereupon rates are as high as 1,4%. Intraoperative ultrasonography (IOUS) seems to be an effective tool in reducing IBDI rates (Machi, 2009 - BDI: 0%, 1381 LCs), but unfortunately there are few studies about this technique, which requires a long learning curve (according to the author, > 100 procedures) discouraging its widespread. As one can infer from Table 1, showing incidences from the total amount of 412585 LCs performed in several international centres, the median estimated incidence is 0,2%, certainly lower than those reported before 2006. Nevertheless, it's difficult to establish if currently this value of incidence is equal to that reported in OCs, sometimes reported as low as 0,1%. In conclusion, according to authors' analysis, it seems that during the last years IBDI incidence following LCs is lower than that reported in the previous fifteen years since the approach was introduced in 1987. This occurrence could be related to the wider experience of the several centres, to the spread of better technologies, and likely a greater concern and a careful sensitivity of surgeons' community toward this issue.

5. Risk factors

Several risk factors are related to IBDI, which can be classified as patient factors, local factors due to illness, and extrinsic factors, related to the surgeon and his operative technique. Patient factors are male gender, advanced age and obesity (Waage, 2006). Local factors include: congenital malformations, such as partial liver agenesis (Fields, 2008); anatomical anomalies of the biliary tract (BT) (Colovic, 2009), concerning both the proximality and the confluence between the cystic duct and the main BT, which may be angular (75%), parallel (20%) or spiral (5%), so jeopardizing its dissection (Strasberg, 2008); inflammatory conditions, such as acute cholecystitis, that increases up to three times the risk of IBDI with a 5% rate, are the most important predisposing factor for IBDI in LC (Kitano, 2002). The reason of this rate is what Strasberg name "hidden cystic duct syndrome", or otherwise "second cystic duct syndrome". When the surgeon dissects the infundibulum to identify the cystic duct as first step (infundibular technique), without first isolating Calot structures, the hepatocholedochus may be confused with a false cystic duct, and sectioned. This misidentification is more likely with acute and chronic inflammation, large stones impacted in the infundibulum, adhesions between gallbladder and choledochus or intrahepatic gallbladder (Chapman, 2003). These last conditions are related to extrinsic factors, too. In fact, when anatomy is not clear, dissective technique must be meticulous. So surgeon must not only isolate infundibulum, but also accurately prepare Calot triangle before cutting any structure, in order to avoid IBDI. In LC they are more proximal, and sometimes associated with vascular injuries, often depending on the right hepatic artery. The incidence of vascular injuries during LC is 61% in the series by Koffron (Koffron, 2001) and 47% in the series by Belghiti (Alves, 2003). It is still controversial the possible influence of the associated vascular lesion on the outcome of the surgical biliary diversion. In LC the learning curve seems to be the most important factor for minimising IBDI rates (Archer, 2001). Even surgeon's tiredness has been implicated as a risk factor for IBDI (Yaghoubian, 2008), as testified by decreased incidence with work hour restrictions.

6. How to prevent IBDI

Principles for a correct technique in laparoscopic approach, for preventing IBDI, were largely described since the beginning of laparoscopic era. Use of a 30° camera, avoiding thermocoagulation near the main BT, a meticulous dissection, an accurate haemostasis and eventually conversion to open surgery, whenever is not possible to figure out clearly the anatomy, all of these represent well-known and precious dogmas (Troidl, 1999). During LC correct identification of the cystic duct can made easier in complex cases by several methods. Routinely intraoperative Cholangiography (Traverso , 2006) can show the whole biliary tract, including any anomaly; it can verify the existence of IBDI, leading quickly to treatment. Many authors state that unfortunately many lesions have already been made at time of the radiological investigation, but nonetheless this represent a meaningful step because an early diagnosis is helpful in the outcome of repair. The critical view technique, described by Strasberg in 1995, consists of the identification of the cystic duct and cystic artery through dissection of the upper border of the Calot triangle along the underside of the gallbladder, thereby exposing the base of the liver. Once this view has been achieved, these two structures will be the only entering the gallbladder. Exposing the inner layer of the subserosa could be useful, further optimising the critical view, either for aberrant ducts or swollen gallbladder (Mirrizzi, 1932). The infundibular technique is based on the identification of the cystic duct where it joins the infundibulum. Some authors still recommend this technique, if routinely assisted by the intraoperative cholangiography. It is currently the most widely used and maybe quickest technique, but it has the drawback of not preventing IBDI because of lacking of the contemporary assessment of cystic duct and main BT (an hot point of the hidden cystic duct syndrome). The Fisher method consists of dissecting the gallbladder from the gallbladder bed starting from the bottom to the infundibulum, as in open surgery. Since cystic artery is ligated at the end of this step, this procedure is more bleeding, thereby more dangerous. The use of intraoperative laparoscopic ultrasound represents another method to prevent IBDI. It is a really interesting diagnostic tool, even if it requires an equipped operating room and highly trained staff. A multicentre study by Machi (Machi, 2009) highlighted his usefulness. However, its advantages are unclear compared to the intraoperative cholangiography, neither they submit a standardized technique. So its effectiveness has to be demonstrated, because it is more expensive than cholangiography, highly operator-dependent and not available in every hospital.

7. Diagnosis

Early diagnosis of IBDI is of primary importance, and decisive as well for the long-term results after treatment. IBDI are noticed intraoperatively only in few cases, often by means of bile leaking, allowing an early repair. Unfortunately, in most cases, at times after days or weeks after intervention, diagnosis is accomplished lately, due to the onset of abdominal pain, fever, jaundice, and septic syndrome. An unusual postoperative course may be a warning sign of IBDI. Postoperative diagnosis must be assessed by clinical exam, lab values (cholestasis) and imaging techniques. Liver function tests after bile duct injury may show cholestasis by the rise of Gamma-Glutamyl Transpeptidase (GGT) and and Alkaline Phosphatase (ALP). However, these tests may often be in the normal range. In patients with biliary stricture or complete occlusion, bilirubin is elevated, while in bile leakage, bilirubin may be normal or only mildly elevated, after absorption of bile from the peritoneal cavity (Lau, 2010). Intraoperative recognition of bile duct injuries and its immediate repair is highly advantageous in preventing serious complications (sepsis) and increase repair success rates (Lohan, 2005). Unfortunately, diagnosis is intraoperative only in 10% to 30% of cases (Lee, 2000), while most of them are recognized postoperatively, with patients sometimes complaining of vague abdominal symptoms, 48h after the intervention (biliary abdominal collections, jaundice, anorexia, elevation of cholestasis and liver enzyme values) (Lillemoe, 2006). Finally, we can have delayed diagnosis for cases that often become more complex and with poor prognosis, recognized after a week to months since intervention, with recurrent cholangitis, obstructive jaundice up to secondary biliary cirrhosis (Sicklick, 2005). Ultrasonography is the first investigation which can show fluid collections and dilatation of the biliary tract, but reveals neither the site and seriousness of the lesion nor a coexisting vascular injury, for what Computed tomography with contrast agent is recommended. Scanning with iminodiacetic acid (HIDA scan) can only diagnose bile leaks. MR-cholangiography is at present a fundamental investigation that allows to identify leaks from small biliary radicals or cystic duct stump, together with the presence of arterial injuries and choledocholithiasis. MR- cholangiography with manganese is an efficient method to reveal IBDI, but series in literature (Khalid, 2001) are few. Cholangiography, both percutaneous transhepatic (PTC) and endoscopic (ERCP), is the gold standard for evaluating bile duct injuries, often essential to plan therapeutic procedure. Sometimes they represent the ultimate treatment. In cases of lesion proximal to the hilum, with either transection or aberrant ducts leaking, ERCP cannot show the biliary tract, so that an anterograde Cholangiography by PTCA is indicated (Pawa, 2009).

8. Management

Management of bile duct injuries is complex and a multidisciplinary approach in tertiary centres is recommended. In any case, early recognition and treatment of septic complications is of paramount importance. Management can be categorized into non-surgical and surgical, and has to be performed in referral centres because often repair intervention represents the only chance of care for the patient. The therapeutic approach and its timing depend on several factors: the extent of lesion, the experience of the surgeon, the inflammatory and haemodynamic status, all of them jeopardize outcome. It is well known that, an intraoperative recognition of the lesion and its immediate repair offers the best long-term results with a low morbidity, reduced hospital stay and costs. The experience of referral hepato-biliary surgery centres plays an important role, as demonstrated by the better success rates of repair (de Reuver, 2007), especially in case of proximal IBDI associated with vascular injury (Bilge, 2003). Non-surgical management is based on endoscopic procedures (ERCP) and on interventional radiology, often mandatory for repair and less expensive. They require bilioenteric continuity. They are less invasive and more appropriate in patients who are not candidates for surgery (Misra, 2004). Recently the development of different types of biliary prostheses contributed hugely to simplify the management of biliary benign strictures (Ramos-De la Medina, 2008). Endoscopic treatment (papillotomy with stenting) is indicated for type A lesions. Its effectiveness decreases if leaks are more proximal, because of differences in the basal or intraductal pressure, of CD length and BT diameter (Marks, 1998). About surgical management, in case of the complete transection of the common hepatic duct or of choledochus, end-to-side Roux-en-Y hepaticojejunostomy represents the best bilio-enteric anastomosis. The defunctionalised loop avoid intestinal reflux into the BT and prevents ascending cholangitis. The hepatoduodenal anastomosis has an increased anastomotic tension and reflux, and a higher rate of developing high debt biliary fistula (Mercado, 2008). Still controversial is the effectiveness and the duration of a transanastomotic tutor, and it depends on surgeon's experience and choice. In case of complete section, an end-to-end anastomosis on T-tube is not indicated because in almost 50% of cases is followed by biliary stricture (Jarnagin, 2009). Biliary diversion should be preferred when vascular damage is expected, even if section of the bile duct is just partial. A T-tube has therefore only a decompressive function and does not act as a tutor for a bilio-biliary hazardous anastomosis; it can therefore be used only in selected cases such as partial section or lesion with a proper vascularisation. Finally, unfortunately, there are some complications that may require liver transplantation: IBDI associated with recurrent episodes of cholangitis, chronic cholestasis and secondary biliary cirrhosis, and lesions of the hepatic hilar vessels, especially the hepatic artery, which according to some authors can lead to an acute hepatic failure (Fernández, 2004), although this occurs rarely in a liver otherwise healthy because of its double blood supply (Stewart, 2004).

9. Hepatico-jejunal anastomosis

A regular evaluation of cholestasis is indicated in patients undergone hepaticojejunostomy, by over ten years lasting follow-up due to the potential onset of long-term complications. The goal of surgical repair of the injured biliary tract is the restoration of a durable bile flow, and the prevention of short- and long-term complications such as biliary fistula, intra-abdominal abscess, and subsequently biliary stricture, recurrent cholangitis, and secondary biliary cirrhosis. A tension-free Roux-en-Y hepaticojejunostomy is the preferred procedure for the majority of bile duct injuries. Tension-free end-to-end anastomoses are rarely possible, even if the duodenum has been largely mobilized. Moreover, a high rate of restricture has been reported for end-to-end repair of laparoscopic bile duct injuries (Stewart, 1995), sometimes up to 100% of cases. For diathermy injury to the bile duct, the anastomosis should be made proximally near to the confluence of the bile ducts to avoid stricture formation, as a consequence to coagulation injury to the collateral network of blood vessels supplying the CBD/CHD (Lau, 2009). Outcome after HJ is evaluated by cholestasis and liver function tests - the clinical presentation of an anastomotic stricture is cholangitis in almost half of the case, and jaundice or abnormal liver function tests in the other half (Goykhman, 2008), with the potential onset of long-term complications (> 10 years) requiring a further intervention, often transhepatic percutaneous stenting. Factors as ischemia, inflammation, and fibrosis may play a fundamental role in the development of strictures. About long-term out come, a poor prognostic factor is serum ALP levels higher than 400 UI six months after intervention (Huang, 2003). Independent poor prognostic factors of the HJ outcome are: surgical repair in the presence of active inflammation (peritonitis), injuries at or above the biliary bifurcation, and bile duct injury with concomitant vascular injury. These factors are associated to a significant higher risk of developing severe biliary complications, such as restrictures, hepatic abscess, and secondary biliary cirrhosis (Schmidt, 2004). Two thirds of recurrences occur within the first two years from the intervention, but stricture recurrence even after 10 years has also been reported (Sutherland, 1999). The long interval from reconstruction to symptomatic late stricture and liver failure underlines the need for long-term follow-up.

10. Conclusions

Analysis of literature related to IBDI following LCs is still difficult and inaccurate, because bile duct injuries are not always standardized, according to the several existing classifications, and as consequence authors do not always specify the type of injury reported. Several papers report laparoscopic techniques with the aim of reducing IBDI, but none of them is absolutely perfect or even better than others, because as a matter of fact IBDI may occur even to the most skilled laparoscopic surgeons. Accordingly, we might suppose that these complications are not exclusively due to unskilfulnes below standards, but they are probably related to the limits of the mininvasive approaches themselves - lack of three-dimensional view and loss of tactile feedback - which could increase operative risks. In other words, compared to a recent pastime, from 1987 to 2005, during which IBDI following LCs had a huge rise, estimated in Italy as high as between 0,3%vs 0,1% (an amount of 300 IBDI per year out of every 90000 LCs), according to the most recent literature a decreasing trend is reported. Everyone must trust in a leading concept: during the first dissective phases, in case of unclarified anatomy, the surgeon must not hesitate about converting, with the aim of carrying out a safer intervention, because of the potential hazard of IBDI. LC is still an ideal approach for symptomatic cholelithiasis, but a cholecystectomy through a "wide subcostal laparotomy" is indicated as well, if preserving from a bile duct injury, which is at present a dreadful complication in terms of morbidity, mortality and social costs. Diffusion and sharing of such principles among surgeons and patients likely represent the most efficient strategy to prevent IBDI. IBDI following LC represent a delicate and interesting chapter in hepato-biliary surgery. They are characterized by high morbidity and sometimes mortality, especially caused by septic complications. The pastime higher incidence seems decreasing and close to that described in traditional surgery, likely due to a better knowledge of the mini-invasive approach and an improved sensitivity toward this issue by the surgical community. Nonetheless they are still causing an increase in healthcare costs because of the investigation, the management and the hospital stay, and moreover for legal issues frustrating to surgeons. Among diagnostic tools, MR Cholangiography is thought to be very important for a suitable biliary-vascular study, but is often followed by second level invasive procedures, that sometimes represent an effective therapeutic option. An early diagnosis is directly related to outcome of the repair, that must be multidisciplinary - endoscopy, interventional radiology, and surgery - in referral centres, because frequently the patient has an unique therapeutic chance. For "major" lesions, Hepaticojejunostomy is the intervention of choice, whereas a T-tube diversion is indicated for selected patients, because of long-term biliary strictures. A regular evaluation of cholestasis is indicated in these cases by means of over ten years follow-up.In case of IBDI, irrespective of biliary repair, the early recognition and treatment of the septic complications, that often rise up mortality, is the most important aim on planning diagnostic and therapeutic work-up.

11. References

Al-Kubati, WR. Bile duct injuries following laparoscopic cholecystectomy: A clinical study. *Saudi Journal of Gastroenterology,* Vol. 16, No. 2, (April - June 2010), pp. 100-104

Alves, A., Farges, O., Nicolet, J.,Watrin, T., Sauvanet, A. & Belghiti, J. Incidence and consequence of an hepatic artery injury in patients with postcholecystectomy bile duct strictures. *Annals of Surgery* , Vol. n.d., No. 238, (2003), pp. 93-96

Archer, SB., Brown, DW., Smith, CD., Branum, GD. & Hunter, JG. Bile duct injury during laparoscopic cholecystectomy: results of a national survey. *Annals of Surgery,* Vol. n.d., No. 234, (2001), pp. 549-558

Avgerinos, C., Kelgiorgi, D., Touloumis, Z., Baltatzi, L. & Dervenis, C. One thousand laparoscopic cholecystectomies in a single surgical unit using the "critical view of safety" technique. *Journal of Gastrointestinal Surgery,* Vol. 13, No. 3, (March 2009), pp. 498-503

Bektas, H., Schrem, H., Winny, M. & Klempnauer, J. Surgical treatment and outcome of iatrogenic bile duct lesions after cholecystectomy and the impact of different clinical classification systems. *British Journal of Surgery,* Vol. n.d., No. 94, (2007), pp. 1119-1127

Bergman, JJ., Van den Brink, GR., Rauws, EA., De Wit, L., Obertop, H., Huibregtse, K., et al. Treatment of bile duct lesions after laparoscopic cholecystectomy. *Gut,* Vol. n.d., No. 38, (1996), pp. 141-147

Bilge, O., Bozkiran, S., Ozden, I., Tekant, Y., Acarli, K., Alper, A. & et al. The effect of concomitant vascular disruption in patients with iatrogenic biliary injuries. *Langenbeck's Archives of Surgery,* Vol. n.d., No. 388, (2003), pp. 265-269

Bismuth, H. (1982) Postoperative strictures of the bile ducts. *The Biliary Tract,* Churchill-Livingstone, New York, NY, pp. 208-209

Boddy, AP., Bennett, JM., Ranka, S. & Rhodes, M. Who should perform laparoscopic cholecystectomy? A 10-year audit. *Surgical Endoscopy*, Vol. 21, No. 9, (September 2007), pp. 1492-1497

Cai, XJ., Gu, XJ., Wang, YF., Yu, H. & Liang, X. Experience in laparoscopic cholecystectomy by exposing common hepatic duct using blunt dissection to prevent bile duct injury. *Zhonghua Yi Xue Za Zhi*, Vol. 87, No. 20, (May 2007), pp. 1425-1426

Chapman, WC., Abecassis, M., Jarnagin, W., Mulvihill, S. & Strasberg, SM. Bile duct injuries 12 years after the introduction of laparoscopic cholecystectomy. *Journal of Gastrointestinal Surgery.* , Vol. n.d., No. 7, (2003), pp. 412-416

Colovic, RB. Isolated segmental, sectoral and right hepatic bile duct injuries. *World Journal of Gastroenterology* , Vol. n.d., No. 15, (2009), pp. 1415-1419

Csendes, A., Navarrete, C., Burdiles, P. & Yarmuch, J. Treatment of common bile duct injuries during laparoscopic cholecystectomy: endoscopic and surgical management. *World Journal of Surgery*, Vol. n.d., No. 25, (2001), pp. nd

de Reuver, PR., Grossmann, I., Busch, OR., Obertop, H., Van Gulik, TM. & Gouma DJ. Referral pattern and timing of repair are risk factors for complications after reconstructive surgery for bile duct injury. *Annals of Surgery.* , Vol. n.d., No. 245, (2007), pp. 763-770

de Reuver, PR., Wind, J., Cremers, JE., Busch, OR., van Gulik, TM. & Gouma, DJ. Litigation after laparoscopic cholecystectomy: an evaluation of the Dutch arbitration system for medical malpractice. *Journal of the American College of Surgeons,* Vol. 206, No. 2, (February 2008), pp. 328-334

de Santibañes, E., Palavecino, M., Ardiles, V. & Pekolj, J. Bile duct injuries: management of late complications. *Surgical Endoscopy*, Vol. 20, No. 11, (November 2006), pp. 1648-1653

Fernández, JA., Robles, R., Marín, C., Sánchez-Bueno, F., Ramírez, P. & Parrilla, P. Laparoscopic iatrogeny of the hepatic hilum as an indication for liver transplantation. *Liver Transplantation.* , Vol. n.d., No. 10, (2004), pp. 147-152

Fields, RC., Heiken, JP. & Strasberg SM. Biliary injury after laparoscopic cholecystectomy in a patient with right liver agenesis: case report and review of the literature. *J Gastrointestinal Surgery*, Vol. n.d., No. 12, (2008), pp. 1577-1581

Frattaroli, FM., Reggio, D., Guadalaxara, A., Illomei, G. & Pappalardo, G. Benign biliary strictures: a review of 21 years of experience. *Journal of the American College of Surgeons.*, Vol. n.d., No. 183, (1996), pp. 506-513

Ghnnam, W., Malek, J., Shebl, E., Elbeshry, T. & Ibrahim, A. Rate of conversion and complications of laparoscopic cholecystectomy in a tertiary care center in Saudi Arabia. *Annals of Saudi Medicine*, Vol. 30, No. 2, (March - April 2010), pp. 145-148

Giger, UF., Michel, JM., Opitz, I., Th Inderbitzin, D., Kocher, T., Krähenbühl, L. & Swiss Association of Laparoscopic and Thoracoscopic Surgery (SALTS) Study Group. Risk factors for perioperative complications in patients undergoing laparoscopic cholecystectomy: analysis of 22,953 consecutive cases from the Swiss Association of Laparoscopic and Thoracoscopic Surgery database. *Journal of the American College of Surgeons*, Vol. 203, No. 5, (November 2006), pp. 723-728

Giger, U., Ouaissi, M., Schmitz, SF., Krähenbühl, S. & Krähenbühl, L. Bile duct injury and use of cholangiography during laparoscopic cholecystectomy. *British Journal of Surgery*, Vol. 98, No. 3, (March 2011), pp. 391-396

Goykhman, Y., Kory, I., Small, R., Kessler, A., Klausner, JM., Nakache, R. & Ben-Haim, M. Long-term Outcome and Risk Factors of Failure after Bile Duct Injury Repair. *Journal of Gastrointestinal Surgery*, Vol. n.d., No. 12, (2008), pp. 1412-1417

Gurusamy, K., Samraj, K., Gluud, C., Wilson, E. & Davidson, BR. Meta-analysis of randomized controlled trials on the safety and effectiveness of early versus delayed laparoscopic cholecystectomy for acute cholecystitis. *British Journal of Surgery*, Vol. 97, No. 2, (February 2010), pp. 141-150

Hamad, MA., Nada, AA., Abdel-Atty, MY. & Kawashti, AS. Major biliary complications in 2,714 cases of laparoscopic cholecystectomy without intraoperative cholangiography: a multicenter retrospective study. *Surgical Endoscopy*, Vol. n.d., No. 8, (June 2011), pp. n.d.

Harboe, KM. & Bardram, L. The quality of cholecystectomy in Denmark: outcome and risk factors for 20,307 patients from the national database. *Surgical Endoscopy*, Vol. 25, No. 5, (May 2011), pp. 1630-1641

Harrison, VL., Dolan, JP., Pham, TH., Diggs, BS., Greenstein, AJ., Sheppard, BC. & Hunter, JG. Bile duct injury after laparoscopic cholecystectomy in hospitals with and without surgical residency programs: is there a difference? *Surgical Endoscopy*, Vol. 25, No. 6, (June 2011), pp. 1969-1974

Hobbs, MS., Mai, Q., Knuiman, MW., Fletcher, DR. & Ridout, SC. Surgeon experience and trends in intraoperative complications in laparoscopic cholecystectomy. *British Journal of Surgery*, Vol. 93, No. 7, (July 2006), pp. 844-853

Huang, CS., Lein, HH., Tai, FC. & Wu, CH. Long-term results of major bile duct injury associated with laparoscopic cholecystectomy. *Surgical Endoscopy*, Vol. n.d., No. 17, (2003), pp. 1362–1367

Hussain, MI. & Khan, AF. Outcome of laparoscopic cholecystectomy in acute and chronic cholecystitis. *Saudi Medical Journal*, Vol. 27, No. 5, (May 2006), pp. 657-660

Ibrahim, S., Tay, KH., Lim, SH., Ravintharan, T. & Tan, NC. Analysis of a structured training programme in laparoscopic cholecystectomy. *Langenbeck's Archives of Surgery*, Vol. 393, No. 6, (November 2008), pp. 943-948

Jarnagin, WR. & Blumgart, LH. Operative repair of bile duct injuries involving the hepatic duct confluence. *Archives Surgery* , Vol. 134, No. 7, (July 1999), pp. 769-775

Kapoor, VK. New classification of acute bile duct injuries. *Hepatobiliary & pancreatic diseases international*, Vol. n.d., No. 7, (2008), pp. 555-556

Karvonen, J., Gullichsen, R., Laine, S., Salminen, P. & Grönroos, JM. Bile duct injuries during laparoscopic cholecystectomy: primary and long-term results from a single institution. *Surgical Endoscopy*, Vol. 21, No. 7, (July 2007), pp. 1069-1073

Keus, F., Gooszen, HG. & van Laarhoven, CJ. Open, small-incision, or laparoscopic cholecystectomy for patients with symptomatic cholecystolithiasis. An overview of Cochrane Hepato-Biliary Group reviews. *Cochrane database of systematic reviews*, Vol. 20, No. 1, (January 2010), pp. n.d.

Khalid, TR., Casillas, VJ., Montalvo, BM., Centeno, R. & Levi, JU. Using MR cholangiopancreatography to evaluate iatrogenic bile duct injury. *AJR. American journal of roentgenology*, Vol. n.d., No. 177, (2001), pp. 1347-1352

Kitano, S., Matsumoto, T., Aramaki, M. & Kawano, K. Laparoscopic cholecystectomy for acute cholecystitis. *Journal of hepato-biliary-pancreatic surgery*, Vol. n.d., No. 9, (2002), pp. 534-537

Koffron, A., Ferrario, M., Parsons, W., Nemcek, A., Saker, M. & Abecassis, M. Failed primary management of iatrogenic biliary injury: incidence and significance of concomitant hepatic arterial disruption. *Surgery* , Vol. n.d., No. 130, (2001), pp. 722-728

Koulas, SG., Tsimoyiannis, J., Koutsourelakis, I., Zikos, N., Pappas-Gogos, G., Siakas, P. & Tsimoyiannis, EC. Laparoscopic cholecystectomy performed by surgical trainees. *JSLS : Journal of the Society of Laparoendoscopic Surgeons / Society of Laparoendoscopic Surgeons*, Vol. 10, No. 4, (October - December 2006), pp. 484-487

Lau, WY. & Lai, EC. Classification of iatrogenic bile duct injury. *Hepatobiliary & pancreatic diseases international*, Vol. n.d., No. 6, (2007), pp. 459-463

Lau, WY., Lai, EC. & Lau, SH. Management of bile duct injury after laparoscopic cholecystectomy: a review. *ANZ Journal of Surgery*, Vol. 80, No. 1-2, (January 2010), pp. 75-81

Ledniczky, G., Fiore, N., Bognár, G., Ondrejka, P. & Grosfeld, JL. Evaluation of perioperative cholangiography in one thousand laparoscopic cholecystectomies. *Chirurgia (Bucur)*, Vol. 101, No. 3, (May - June 2006), pp. 267-272

Lee, CM., Stewart, L. & Way, LW. Postcholecystectomy abdominal bile collections. *Archives of Surgery* , Vol. 135, No. 5, (2000), pp. 538-544

Lien, HH., Huang, CC., Liu, JS., Shi, MY., Chen, DF., Wang, NY., Tai, FC. & Huang, CS. System approach to prevent common bile duct injury and enhance performance of laparoscopic cholecystectomy. *Surgical laparoscopy, endoscopy & percutaneous techniques*, Vol. 17, No. 3, (June 2007), pp. 164-170

Lillemoe, KD. Evaluation of suspected bile duct injuries. *Surgical Endoscopy*, Vol. n.d., No. 20, (2006), pp. 1638-1643

Lohan, D., Walsh, S., McLoughlin, R. & et al. Imaging of the complications of laparoscopic cholecystectomy. *European Radiology*, Vol. 15, No. 5, (2005), pp. 904-912

Machi, J., Johnson, JO., Deziel, DJ., Soper, NJ., Berber, E., Siperstein, A., Hata, M., Patel, A., Singh, K. & Arregui, ME. The routine use of laparoscopic ultrasound decreases bile duct injury: a multicenter study. *Surgical Endoscopy*, Vol. 23, No. 2, (February 2009), pp. 384-388

Malik, AM., Laghari, AA., Talpur, AH. & Khan, A. Iatrogenic biliary injuries during laparoscopic cholecystectomy. A continuing threat. *International journal of surgery*, Vol. 6, No. 5, (October 2008), pp. 392-395

Marakis, GN., Pavlidis, TE., Ballas, K., Aimoniotou, E., Psarras, K., Karvounaris, D., Rafailidis, S., Demertzidis, H. & Sakantamis, AK. Major complications during laparoscopic cholecystectomy. *International journal of surgery*, Vol. 92, No. 3, (May - June 2007), pp. 142-146

Marks, JM., Ponsky, JL., Shillingstad, RB. & Singh, J. Biliary stenting is more effective than sphincterotomy in the resolution of biliary leaks. *Surgical Endoscopy*, Vol. n.d., No. 12, (1998), pp. 327-330

McMahon, AJ., Fullarton, G., Baxter, JN. & O'Dwyer, PJ. Bile duct injury and bile leakage in laparoscopic cholecystectomy. *British Journal of Surgery*, Vol. n.d., No. 82, (1995), pp. 307-313

Mercado, MA., Chan, C., Salgado-Nesme, N. & López-Rosales, F. Intrahepatic repair of bile duct injuries. A comparative study. *Journal of Gastrointestinal Surgery*, Vol. n.d., No. 12, (2008), pp. 364-368

Mirrizzi, PL. La cholangiografía durante las operaciones de las vías biliares. *Boletines y trabajos - Sociedad de Cirugía de Buenos Aires*, Vol. n.d., No. 16, (1932), pp. 1133

Misra, S., Melton, GB., Geschwind, JF., Venbrux, AC., Cameron, JL. & Lillemoe, KD. Percutaneous management of bile duct strictures and injuries associated with laparoscopic cholecystectomy: a decade of experience. *Journal of the American College of Surgeons*, Vol. n.d., No. 198, (2004), pp. 218-226

Neuhaus, P., Schmidt, SC., Hintze, RE., Adler, A., Veltzke, W., Raakow, R., et al. Classification and treatment of bile duct injuries after laparoscopic cholecystectomy. *Chirurg*, Vol. n.d., No. 71, (2000), pp. 166-173

Nickkholgh, A., Soltaniyekta, S. & Kalbasi, H. Routine versus selective intraoperative cholangiography during laparoscopic cholecystectomy: a survey of 2,130 patients undergoing laparoscopic cholecystectomy. *Surgical Endoscopy*, Vol. 20, No. 6, (June 2006), pp. 868-874

National Institute of Health (NIH) Consensus conference. Gallstones and laparoscopic cholecystectomy. *Journal of the American Medical Association*, Vol. 269, No. 8, (1993), pp. 1018-1024

Nuzzo, G. (2002). Le lesioni della via biliare principale. Relazione biennale Atti congresso nazionale S.I.C., Rome, October 2002

Nuzzo, G., Giuliante, F., Giovannini, I., Ardito, F., D'Acapito, F., Vellone, M., Murazio, M. & Capelli, G. Bile duct injury during laparoscopic cholecystectomy: results of an Italian national survey on 56 591 cholecystectomies. *Archives of Surgery*, Vol. 140, No. 10, (October 2005), pp. 986-992

Pawa, S. & Al-Kawas, FH. ERCP in the management of biliary complications after cholecystectomy. *Curr Gastroenterol Rep.*, Vol. n.d., No. 11, (2009), pp. 160-166

Pfluke, JM. & Bowers, SP. Jr. Laparoscopic intraoperative biliary ultrasonography: findings during laparoscopic cholecystectomy for acute disease. *J Laparoendosc Adv Surg Tech A*, Vol. 21, No. 6, (July - August 2011), pp. 505-509

Plummer, JM., Mitchell, DI., Duncan, ND., McDonald, AH. & Arthurs, M. Bile duct injuries in the laparoscopic era: the University Hospital of the West Indies experience. *West Indian Med J.*, Vol. 55, No. 4, (September 2006), pp. 228-231

Priego, P., Ramiro, C., Molina, JM., Rodríguez Velasco, G., Lobo, E., Galindo, J. & Fresneda, V. Results of laparoscopic cholecystectomy in a third-level university hospital after 17 years of experience. *Rev Esp Enferm Dig*, Vol. 101, No. 1, (January 20109), pp. 20-30

Ramos-De la Medina, A., Misra, S., Leroy, AJ. & Sarr, MG. Management of benign biliary strictures by percutaneous interventional radiologic techniques (PIRT). *HPB(Oxford)*, Vol. n.d., No. 10, (2008), pp. 428-432

Sanjay, P., Kulli, C., Polignano, F. & Tait, I. Optimal surgical technique, use of intra-operativecholangiography and management of acute gallbladder disease: the results of a nationwide survey in the UK and Ireland. *Ann R Coll Surg Engl*, Vol. n.d., No. n.d., (2010), pp. n.d.

Sarli, L., Costi, R. & Roncoroni, L. Intraoperative cholangiography and bile duct injury. *Surgical Endoscopy*, Vol. 20, No. 1, (January 2006), pp. 176-177

Schmidt, SC., Langrehr, JM., Hintze, RE. & Neuhaus, P. Long-term results and risk factors influencing outcome of major bile duct injuries following cholecystectomy. *British Journal of Surgery*, Vol. 92, No. n.d., (2005), pp. 76-82

Shea, JA., Healey, MJ., Berlin, JA., Clarke, JR., Malet, PF., Staroscik, RN., et al. Mortality and complications associated with laparoscopic cholecystectomy. A meta-analysis. *Annals of Surgery* Vol. 224, No. 5, (1996), pp. 609-620

Sicklick, JK., Camp, MS., Lillemoe, KD. & et al. Surgical management of bile duct injuries sustained during laparoscopic cholecystectomy: perioperative results in 200 patients. Proceedings of the 116th Annual Meeting of the Southern Surgical Association. December 2004. *Ann Surg* , Vol. 241, No. 5, (2005), pp. 786-792

Siewert, JR., Ungeheuer, A. & Feussner, H. Bile duct lesions in laparoscopic cholecystectomy. *Chirurg*, Vol. n.d., No. 65, (1994), pp. 748-757

Stanisić, V., Bakić, M., Magdelinić ,M., Kolasinac, H., Vlaović, D. & Stijović, B. A prospective evaluation of laparoscopic cholecystectomy in the treatment of chronic cholelithiasis - a five-year experience. *Med Pregl*, Vol. 64, No. 1-2, (January - February 2011), pp. 77-83

Stewart, L. & Way, LW. Bile duct injuries during laparoscopic cholecystectomy. Factors that influence the results of treatment. *Arch. Surg*, Vol. n.d., No. 130, (1995), pp. 1123-1128

Stewart, L., Robinson, TN., Lee, CM. et al. Right hepatic artery injury associated with laparoscopic bile duct injury: incidence, mechanism, and consequences. *J Gastrointest Surg*, Vol. 8, No. 5, (2004), pp. 523-530

Stewart, L., Robinson, TN., Lee, CM., Liu, K., Whang, K. & Way, W. Right hepatic artery injury associated with laparoscopic bile duct injury: incidence, mechanism, and consequences. *J Gastrointest Surg.* , Vol. n.d., No. 8, (2004), pp. 523-530

Strasberg, SM., Hertl, M. & Soper, NJ. An analysis of the problem of biliary injury during laparoscopic cholecystectomy. *Journal of the American College of Surgeons*, Vol. n.d., No. 180, (1995), pp. 101-125

Strasberg, SM. Error traps and vasculo-biliary injury in laparoscopic and open cholecystectomy. *J Hepatobiliary Pancreat Surg*, Vol. n.d., No. 15, (2008), pp. 284-292

Strasberg, SM. & Brunt, LM. Rationale and use of the critical view of safety in laparoscopic cholecystectomy. *J Am Coll Surg*, Vol. 211, No. n.d., (2010), pp. 132–138

Sutherland, F., Launois, B., Staescu, M., Campion, JP., Spiliopoulos, Y. & Stasik, C. A refined approach to the repair of postcholecystectomy bile duct strictures. *Arch Surg*, Vol. n.d., No. 134, (1999), pp. 299-302

Tan, JT., Suyapto, DR., Neo, EL. & Leong, PS. Prospective audit of laparoscopic cholecystectomy experience at a secondary referral centre in South australia. *ANZ J Surg*, Vol. 76, No. 5, (May 2006), pp. 335-338

Tantia, O., Jain, M., Khanna, S. & Sen, B. Iatrogenic biliary injury: 13,305 cholecystectomies experienced by a single surgical team over more than 13 years. *Surgical Endoscopy*, Vol. 22, No. 4, (April 2008), pp. 1077-1086

Traverso, LW. Intraoperative cholangiography lowers the risk of bile duct injury during cholecystectomy. *Surgical Endoscopy*, Vol. n.d., No. 20, (2006), pp. 1659-1661

Triantafyllidis, I., Nikoloudis, N., Sapidis, N., Chrissidou, M., Kalaitsidou, I. & Chrissidis, T. Complications of laparoscopic cholecystectomy: our experience in a district general hospital. *Surg Laparosc Endosc Percutan Tech*, Vol. 19, No. 6, (December 2009), pp. 449-458

Troidl, H. Disasters of endoscopic surgery and how to avoid them: error analysis. *World J Surg*, Vol. n.d., No. 23, (1999), pp. 846-855

Veen, EJ., Bik, M., Janssen-Heijnen, ML., De Jongh, M. & Roukema, AJ. Outcome measurement in laparoscopic cholecystectomy by using a prospective complication registry: results of an audit. *Int J Qual Health Care*, Vol. 20, No. 2, (April 2008), pp. 144-151

Velanovich, V., Morton, JM., McDonald, M., Orlando, R. 3rd, Maupin, G., Traverso, LW. SAGES Outcomes Committee. Analysis of the SAGES outcomes initiative cholecystectomy registry. *Surgical Endoscopy*, Vol. 20, No. 1, (January 2006), pp. 43-50

Waage, A. & Nilsson M. Iatrogenic bile duct injury: a populationbased study of 152 776 cholecystectomies in the Swedish Inpatient Registry. *Arch Surg.* , Vol. n.d., No. 141, (2006), pp. 1207-1213

Wenner, DE., Whitwam, P., Turner, D., Chadha & A., Degani, J. Laparoscopic cholecystectomy and management of biliary tract stones in a freestanding ambulatory surgery center. *JSLS*, Vol. 10, No. 1, (January - March 2006), pp. 47-51

Yaghoubian, A., Saltmarsh, G., Rosing, DK., Lewis, RJ., Stabile, BE. & de Virgilio, C. Decreased bile duct injury rate during laparoscopic cholecystectomy in the era of the 80-hour resident workweek. *Archives of Surgery*, Vol. 143, No. 9, (September 2008), pp. 847-851

Yamashita, Y., Kimura, T. & Matsumoto, S. A safe laparoscopic cholecystectomy depends upon the establishment of a critical view of safety. *Surgery Today*, Vol. 40, No. 6, (June 2010), pp. 507-513

Yegiyants, S. & Collins, JC. Operative strategy can reduce the incidence of major bile duct injury in laparoscopic cholecystectomy. *American Surgeon*. Vol. 74, No. 10, (October 2008), pp. 985-987

Yüksel, O., Salman, B., Yilmaz, U., Akyürek, N. & Tatlicioğlu, E. Timing of laparoscopic cholecystectomy for subacute calculous cholecystitis: early or interval--a prospective study. *Journal of Hepatobiliary and pancreatic Surgery.*, Vol. 13, No. 5, (2006), pp. 421-426

3

Expression and Function of Renal Organic Anion Transporters in Cholestasis

Anabel Brandoni and Adriana Mónica Torres
Area Farmacología. Facultad de Ciencias Bioquímicas y Farmacéuticas
Universidad Nacional de Rosario
Argentina

1. Introduction

Acute jaundice due to bile duct obstruction is defined as the retention of bile and bile components. Kidney and liver are largely responsible for inactivation and excretion of drugs, including organic anions, and other chemicals. In obstructive jaundice, adaptive mechanisms may permit urinary excretion of those potentially toxic compounds that could not be eliminated by the liver because biliary transport is impaired (Reichen & Simon, 1988; Klaassen & Aleksunes, 2010; Hagenbuch 2010).

A large and diverse number of organic, or weak organic acids that exist as anions at physiological pH, are secreted by mammalian renal tubules principally along the proximal portion of the nephron. Although this system secretes a number of endogenous compounds, it is generally accepted that is particularly important in secreting numerous exogenous compounds, including pharmacologically active substances, industrial and environmental toxins, and plant and animal toxins (Wright & Dantzler, 2004; G. Burckhardt & Pritchard, 2000). The renal organic anion transport plays a critical role, in protecting against the toxic effects of these anionic substances, by removing them from the blood principally via the organic anion transport mechanisms found in the apical and basolateral membrane of renal epithelial cells. Several carrier proteins have been cloned and are functionally characterized from both membrane domains of rat kidneys (El-Sheikh et al., 2008; Wright & Dantzler, 2004). Defining the modifications on the expression of these transporters is important, both to understand the cholestatic process and to identify potential therapeutic targets.

Cholestasis has been shown to alter the transport of bile salts and other organic anions (Denk et al., 2004; Klaassen & Aleksunes, 2010). The modulation in the expression of renal organic anion transporters constitutes a compensative mechanism to overcome the hepatic dysfunction in the elimination of organic anions.

This chapter reviews our current knowledge of the significant roles played by these transporters in organic anions elimination, focusing particularly in their renal expression and in the mechanisms involved in the regulation of their expression and function in extrahepatic cholestasis.

2. Organic anion transporters

The expression and function of several organic anion transporters in kidneys from rats with obstructive cholestasis will be reviewed. These transport proteins are listed below:

- Organic Anion Transporter 1 (Oat1)
- Organic Anion Transporter 3 (Oat3)
- Bilitranslocase (BTL)
- BSP/Bilirubin Binding Protein (BBBP)
- Sodium dependent Bile Salt Transporter (ASBT)
- Organic Anion Transporting Polipeptide 1 (Oatp1)
- Multidrug Resistance Protein 2 (Mrp2)

Oat1, Oat3, BTL and BBBP are expressed in the basolateral membranes. BBBP is also expressed in apical membrane, together with ASBT, Oatp1 and Mrp2. Their membrane localization is shown in Figure 1.

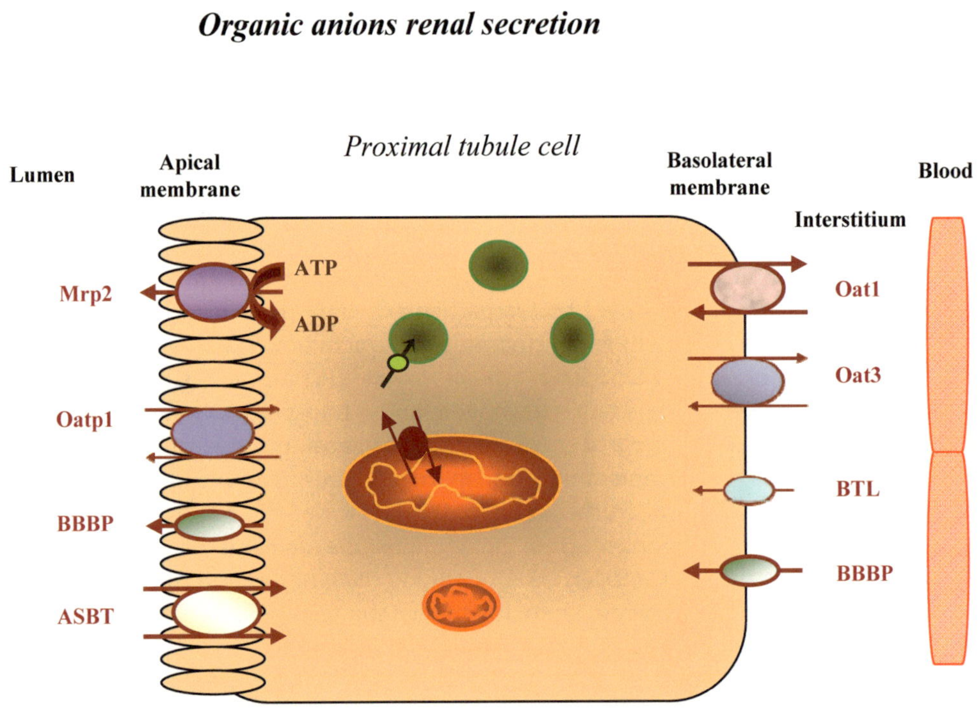

Fig. 1. Organic anion transporters in proximal renal tubule cell. For proteins abbreviations see the text.

2.1 Oat1

Organic anion transporter 1 (Oat1) is a key organic anions/α-ketoglutarate exchanger in the energetically linked basolateral entry of organic anions into the proximal tubule cells of the kidneys (Tojo et al., 1999; Kojima et al., 2002). Its substrate selectivity is markedly broad.

Oat1 is expressed predominantly in the kidneys and weakly in the brain. Oat1 couples organic anions entry to dicarboxylate exit (Sweet, 2005; Torres et al., 2008; Brandoni & Torres, 2010; G. Burckhardt & B.C. Burckhardt, 2011). This protein has been immunolocalized to the basolateral surface of the proximal tubule. Oat1 mediates the transport of many compounds (dicarboxylates, nucleotides, prostaglandins, antivirals, loop and thiazide diuretics, β-lactam antibiotics, non-steroidal anti-inflammatory drugs, including the prototypical substrate of the classical pathway, para-aminohippurate (PAH) (Brandoni & Torres, 2010; G. Burckhardt & B.C. Burckhardt, 2011). This has been demonstrated *in vitro* by its heterologously expression following microinjection of Oat1 cRNA into *Xenopus* oocytes or transfection of Oat1 cDNA into epithelial cell lines (B.C. Burckhardt & G. Burckhardt, 2003; Russel et al., 2002; Van Wert et al., 2010). Eraly *et al.* (2006) have generated a colony of Oat1 knockout mice, permitting the elucidation of the role of Oat1 in the context of other potentially functional redundant transporters. They found that the knockout mice manifest a profound loss of organic anion transport (e.g. PAH) both *ex vivo* (in isolated renal slices) as well as *in vivo* (as indicated by loss of renal secretion). In the case of the organic anion, furosemide, loss of renal secretion in knockout animals resulted in impaired diuretic responsiveness to this drug (Eraly et al., 2006). These results indicate an important role for Oat1 transporter in the handling of organic anions by the classical pathway.

Connected to this, we have reported an up regulation of Oat1 protein expression in rats with an early phase of acute obstructive cholestasis which might explain the increased renal elimination of the well-known organic anions, PAH and furosemide (FS) (Brandoni et al., 2006a). Performing bile duct ligation (BDL) as a well-established model of cholestasis (Brandoni & Torres, 2009a), we have determined an increase in the systemic clearance of PAH associated to an increase in the abundance of Oat1 in renal cortex homogenates in rats at 21 h after bile duct ligation (early phase of acute extrahepatic cholestasis) (Brandoni et al., 2003a).

FS is a well-known loop diuretic secreted through the organic anion transport system. The capacity of the organic anion transport system to secrete a diuretic determines its intraluminal concentration, which is critical for a diuretic activity. Oat1 and Oat3 are involved in the renal tubular secretion of FS and are thereby responsible for their delivery to the site of action in effective amounts (Hasannejad et al., 2004; G. Burckhardt & B.C. Burckhardt, 2011). The protein expression of Oat1 was significantly increased both in cortical homogenates and in basolateral membranes from kidneys after 21 hours of BDL (Brandoni et al., 2006a; Brandoni et al., 2003a). This Oat1 up regulation might lead to a higher elimination of its transported compounds. In fact, we found that systemic clearance and urinary excretion of PAH were both higher in BDL rats. Connected to this, PAH uptake rate (Brandoni et al., 2006a) was increased in basolateral membranes vesicles from BDL rats showing a higher Vmax than Sham animals and no difference in Km. Moreover, Oat1 up-regulation was associated with a concomitant increase of systemic and renal FS clearance.

Similar studies were performed by Brandoni *et al.* (Brandoni et al., 2006b) after 3 days of bile duct ligation (the peak of elevation of serum bile acids and bilirubin). After this time, BDL rats displayed a reduction in the renal elimination of PAH. Oat1 protein expression in kidney homogenates was not modified, but decreased in basolateral membranes. This study demonstrated, once more, the key role of Oat1 expression in the impaired elimination of

PAH after 3 days of obstructive cholestasis. So, the evolution time of obstructive cholestasis has an important impact in the regulation of Oat1.

It has been described that protein kinase C (PKC) induces Oat1 down-regulation through carrier retrieval from the cell membrane. Various humoral factors induced by 3 days of bile duct ligation may probably lead to the activation of PKC. Moreover, bile acids and high bilirubin levels can activate PKC (G. Burckhardt & B.C. Burckhardt, 2011; Hirohata et al., 2002). It has been demonstrated that 3 days of bile duct ligation is the period in which serum bile acids and bilirubin levels reach the peak of elevation. We therefore postulate that the peak of elevation of bile acids and bilirubin can also trigger PKC activation. This PKC activation may cause the phosphorylation of caveolin-2, which may induce internalization of caveolae with Oat1 protein anchored with caveolin as has been recently suggested by Kwak *et. al.* (2005).

In summary, in this experimental model during an early phase of acute extrahepatic cholestasis where no evident renal cell injury exists yet, an Oat1 up regulation connected with an increase in renal organic anion elimination was demonstrated. The protein expression of Oat1 was significantly increased both in cortical homogenates and in basolateral membranes from kidneys after 21 hours of BDL, which might suggest an increase in the synthesis or a decrease in the degradation of this membrane transporter. In this model, Oat1 up regulation might be found in order to enhance renal secretion of toxic compounds that may be harmful in the presence of the pathological state. Connected to this, Tanaka *et al.* (2002) found that bilirubin ditaurate, sulfate conjugated bile acids, and some components of the human bile up regulate the expression of Mrp2 in human renal tubular cells. On the other hand, we found an increased ^{3}H-PAH uptake by S2 cells expressing Oat1 in the presence of bilirubin ditaurate (Brandoni et al., 2006c).

Contrary to what has been observed during an early phase of acute extrahepatic cholestasis, Oat1 expression significantly decreased in the basolateral membranes from kidneys after 3 days of bile duct ligation (Brandoni et al., 2006b). It has been suggested an internalization of membrane transporters or an inhibition in the recruitment of preformed transporters into the membranes. This study stressed, once more, the critical role of Oat1 renal expression in the excretion of PAH, in a model of extrahepatic cholestasis in rats.

2.2 Oat3

Oat3 is mainly expressed in kidneys, and to a lesser extent in brain and liver. The human Oat3 gene is paired with that of Oat1 and located on chromosome 11q12.3. Inmunohistochemistry revealed the location of Oat3 at the basolateral membrane of renal proximal tubules (Cha et al., 2001; Kojima et al., 2002). In rats, Oat3 was also found in several other nephron segments including the thick ascending limb of Henle's loop, distal convoluted tubule and collecting ducts. Oat3 is the predominant organic anion transporter in the human kidney. Oat3 has a broad spectrum of substrates, and it mediates the transport of PAH, ochratoxin A, estrone sulfate (ES), cimetidine, benzylpenicillin, cephaloridine and glutarate. The selectivity of Oat3 overlaps that of Oat1, but affinities for several substrates appear to permit discrimination between both transporters. For example, Oat3 displays a moderately high affinity for ES, whereas Oat1 interacts little with ES (Sweet, 2005; Brandoni & Torres, 2010; Torres et al., 2008; Burckhardt & Burckhardt, 2011). Consequently, ES has been frequently used as a test substrate for Oat3 activity. Oat3 can operate as an organic anion/dicarboxylate exchanger (Sweet et al., 2003, Bakhiya et al., 2003). Recent experiments with tissue from Oat3 knockout mice show reduced uptake of PAH, ES, and taurocholate in renal cortical slices and nearly complete inhibition of transport of the fluorescent organic anion fluorescein in intact choroid plexus (Sweet et al., 2002).

Brandoni *et al* (2003a, 2006a) have studied the cortical renal expression of Oat3 in association with the pharmacokinetics and renal excretion of PAH and FS in rats with acute extrahepatic cholestasis. Male Wistar rats underwent bile duct ligation (BDL rats). All studies were carried out 21 h after surgery. The systemic and renal clearance of both PAH and FS increased in BDL rats. In kidneys from BDL rats, immunoblotting showed a significant increase in the abundance of both Oat1 (as described above) and Oat3 in homogenates from renal cortex. In basolateral membranes from the kidney cortex of BDL rats, Oat1 abundance was also increased and Oat3 abundance was not modified. Immunohistochemical techniques confirmed these results. Acute obstructive jaundice is associated with an upregulation of Oat1 and Oat3, which might explain, at least in part, the increased systemic and renal elimination of PAH and FS. In this connection, extrahepatic cholestasis is associated with the production of various cytokines and growth factors that may affect gene transcription (Plebani et al., 1999).

Three days of BDL is the period in which serum bile acids and bilirubin levels reach the peak of elevation (Tanaka et al., 2002; Lee et al., 2001; Pei et al., 2002). Brandoni *et al* (2006b) have studied Oat1 as previously described and also Oat3 function and expression after 3 days of BDL. After this time, BDL rats displayed a reduction in the renal elimination of PAH. Oat1 protein expression in kidney homogenates was not modified, but it decreased in the basolateral membranes. On the contrary, Oat3 expression increased both in homogenates and basolateral membranes from kidneys after three days of BDL. Oat3 is found in various cells and in all parts of the nephron, whereas Oat1 is confined to proximal tubules (Kojima et al., 2002). The human and rat Oat3 transport PAH with relatively high affinity (87 µmol/L and 65 µmol/L respectively) (Wright & Dantzler, 2004; Anzai et al., 2006; Rizwan & Burckhardt, 2007; Cha et al., 2002), similarly to Oat1. On the contrary, ES, cholate, and taurocholate are substrates for Oat3 and not for Oat1 using *in vivo* and *in vitro* methodologies (Wright & Dantzler, 2004; Anzai et al., 2006; Rizwan & Burckhardt, 2007; Eraly et al., 2006; Cha et al., 2002; Sweet et al., 2002). The over-expression of Oat3 does not compensate for the down-regulation of Oat1 regarding PAH transport because in this disease the high plasma levels of bile acids compete with PAH for Oat3 transport (Brandoni et al., 2006 b; Torres, 2008). Moreover, bile acids regulate the expression of several genes involved in bile salt transport (Rost et al., 2003; Boyer et al., 2006). It is possible that high bile acid levels up-regulate Oat3 expression without affecting Oat1 expression; being this another example of substrate specific regulation.

Chen et al. (2008) have demonstrated that Oat3 is responsible for renal secretion of bile acids during cholestasis and that the pharmacokinetic profile of Oat3 substrates may be affected by cholestasis. In obstructive cholestasis, the main route to excrete bile acids is urinary excretion. It has been demonstrated that Oat3 protein expression level is increased in Eisai hyperbilirubinemic rats (EHBR). EHBR are mutant without multidrug resistance-associated protein 2 that show higher serum and urinary concentration of bile acids, compared with Sprague-Dawley (SD) rats (wild type). On the contrary, the expression of Oat1 was unchanged. Moreover, the transport activities of rat and human Oat3, but not Oat1 were markedly inhibited by various bile acids such as chenodeoxycholic acid and cholic acid. Cholic acid, glycocholic acid and taurocholic acid, which mainly increased during cholestasis are transported by Oat3 (Chen et al., 2008; Burckhardt and Burckhardt, 2011). These authors also demonstrated that the plasma concentration of cefotiam, a specific substrate for Oat3, was more increased in EHBR than in SD rats despite upregulation of Oat3·. This may be due to the competitive inhibition of cefotiam transport by bile acids via Oat3. These results suggested that renal Oat3 but not Oat1 plays critical roles in the adaptative responses to the renal handling of bile acids in cholestasis.

In summary, these findings indicate that Oat3 plays an important pathophysiological role in protecting tissues from cholestatic injury by stimulating the renal secretion of bile acids. From a pharmacokinetic standpoint, it is possible that increased serum bile acids and/or administration of ursodeoxycholic acid (UDCA), recently introduced for cholestatic liver disease therapy (Paumgartner & Beuers, 2004) could influence the tubular secretion of anionic drugs via Oat3 as was demonstrated for cefotiam. So, in this situation, more attention should be paid to prevent the occurrence of drug interaction or drug-induced toxicity.

2.3 BTL

The membrane protein bilitranslocase (BTL) is not a bile acid transporter, but rather a bile pigment transporter that was originally isolated from rat livers (Tiribelli et al, 1978; Passamonti et al. 2009). Bilitranslocase has been indicated as the protein responsible for the electrogenic hepatic uptake of cholephilic organic anions, such as bromosulfophtalein (BSP) and thymol blue, the tetrapyrrole bilirubin, and flavonoids (the anthocyanin malvidin 3-glucoside and the flavonol quercetin) (Passamonti et al. 2009). Bilitranslocase has also been detected in basolateral plasma membranes from kidney cells and it has been demonstrated to be involved in the renal transport of BSP, bilirubin and anthocyanins (Elías et al., 1990; Vanzo et al., 2008). In this way, bilitranslocase contributes to the hepatic and renal elimination of exogenous organic anions (such as BSP), endogenous metabolites (such as bilirubin) and anthocyanins (flavonoid-based pigments that are present in many fruits and vegetables in the human diet, which have been reported to be positively implicated in human health (Vanzo et al., 2008; Passamonti et al. 2009)).

To evaluate the functional activity of bilitranslocase, we measured BSP electrogenic uptake in liver plasma membrane and in renal basolateral membrane vesicles prepared from sham and BDL rats (Brandoni et al., 2010). No modifications were observed in bilitranslocase activity and in the abundance in liver plasma membrane vesicles from BDL rats. On the contrary, extrahepatic cholestasis resulted in a marked increase of renal BSP uptake and this was due to an important increase in V_{max} (capacity). The capacity of a transfer is principally determined by the total number of active carriers presented in renal basolateral membrane vesicles. The difference in V_{max} indicates that a higher number of functional carrier units exists in renal basolateral membrane vesicles from BDL rats, which is in agreement with the higher expression of bilitranslocase in basolateral membranes. The observation that BDL rats have a higher renal expression of bilitranslocase at the basolateral membranes despite no change in this protein abundance in kidney homogenates suggests an alteration in bilitranslocase trafficking that might be caused by an increased recruitment of preformed transporters into the membranes or an inhibition in the internalization of membrane transporters.

These results suggest that the complex series of hormonal changes induced in kidneys by extrahepatic cholestasis (Sheen et al., 2010) might influence the regulation of bilitranslocase and Oatp1 in a similar way. The characteristic accumulation of bile acids, bilirubin, and other potential toxins in cholestasis may affect transcriptional and posttranscriptional regulatory mechanisms (Donner et al., 2007; Geier et al., 2007). In this connection, as it has been mentioned earlier, bilirubin, sulfate-conjugated bile acid and human bile up regulated the expression of Mrp2 in renal tubular cells but not in liver cells (Tanaka et al., 2002).

In summary, the higher renal expression and function of bilitranslocase in renal basolateral membranes from rats with obstructive cholestasis might also contribute to the dramatic increase in BSP renal excretion observed in this experimental model. This would be another compensation mechanism to overcome the hepatic dysfunction in the elimination of organic anions.

2.4 BBBP

BSP/Bilirubin binding protein (BBBP) is a protein isolated from rat liver located on the sinusoidal membrane of the liver and described as a transport protein involved in the well known sodium-independent hepatic uptake of BSP and bilirubin (Stremmel & Berk, 1986; Stremmel et al., 1986; Torres et al., 1993; Torres, 1997). The transport of this protein is electroneutral as indicated by experiments in liver plasma membrane vesicles. BBBP is an organic anion carrier protein expressed in both apical and basolateral membranes from rat kidney cells, which accounts at least in part, for the renal tubular transport of PAH (Torres et al. 2003).

Brandoni et al. (2003b; 2004a; 2004b) have described an increment in BBBP expression in homogenates and in basolateral membranes from kidney cortex after 21 h of obstructive cholestasis without modifications in its apical membrane expression. The increase in BBBP homogenate expression suggests an increment in its synthesis or a decrease in its degradation, while the traffic protein is preferably directed to the basolateral domain. The higher basolateral membrane expression of BBBP could contribute to the higher BSP and PAH renal excretion described in this experimental model of acute cholestasis (Brandoni et al., 2003b; Brandoni et al., 2004a; Brandoni et al., 2004b).

In summary, modifications in hepatic excretion of organic anions have been demonstrated in rats with extrahepatic cholestasis. We have evaluated, in rats with acute bile duct ligation, the urinary excretion of two different organic anions, PAH mainly excreted by the kidneys and BSP mainly excreted by the liver.

The higher abundance of the organic anions carrier BBBP, detected in rats with obstructive jaundice might explain, at least in part, the higher renal capacity to eliminate distinct negatively charge compounds in this group of rats. These results suggest a relevant role of this kind of transporters in renal elimination of those organic anions excreted mainly by liver, in the presence of the obstructive cholestasis.

2.5 ASBT

The sodium dependent bile salt transporter (ASBT) is expressed in the ileum, the apical membrane of cholangiocytes and in the brush border membrane of proximal tubular cells (Christie et al., 1996; Lazaridis et al., 1997; Wilson et al. 1981; Burckhardt et al. 1987).

Bile acids, after secretion with the bile into the small intestine, are nearly completely reabsorbed in the terminal ileum. They return with the portal venous blood to the liver where they are taken up and resecreted into the bile. Some 10-50 % of the reabsorbed bile acids (depending on the bile acid species) escape hepatic uptake and spill over in the peripheral circulation. About 10-30 % of the bile acids, presents in the blood plasma, is not protein-bound and hence is subject to glomerular filtration (Rudman & Kendall, 1957). However, urinary excretion of bile acids is much smaller than the amount filtered due to a nearly complete tubular reabsorption of the filtered bile acids (Weiner et al., 1964; Barnes et al. 1977). Thus, the kidneys also take part in the recirculation process and aid to conserve bile acids. Tubular reabsorption of bile acids is accomplished by ASBT (Wilson et al. 1981; Burckhardt et al. 1987).

After a 14 day bile duct obstruction, a decreased taurocholate transport of brush border membrane vesicles derived from rat kidneys has been found by Lee et al. (2001). The reduced taurocholate uptake was associated with a reduction of renal ABST protein expression in membrane-rich microsomal fractions prepared from rat kidneys.

Schlattjan et al. (2003) have demonstrated that as early as 1 day after induction of an obstructive cholestasis a reduced taurocholate transport of proximal tubular cells can occur without a change in the amount of the transport protein in these cells. The diminished taurocholate transport in this early phase of cholestasis may be mediated by a change of the phosphorylation status and hence activity of ASBT and/or by a redistribution of the transporter between the plasma membrane and intracellular compartments of the proximal tubular cells.

In summary, these studies have demonstrated that there is a functional adaptive down regulation of renal tubular bile acid transport enhancing renal clearance of bile acids during the early phase of an obstructive cholestasis.

2.6 Oatp1

Organic anion-transporting polypeptides (Oatp) are a group of membrane solute carriers with a wide spectrum of amphipathic transport substrates. Several members of the Oatp family are located in the apical membrane of proximal tubules, and have been suggested to play a role in the secretion/reabsorption of selected anionic substrates (Hagenbuch & Meier, 2003; Kalliokoski & Niemi, 2009; Hagenbuch 2010).

The first member of the Oatp gene family of membrane transporters, Oatp1, has been isolated from rat liver and shown to mediate Na^+-independent saturable transport of BSP (Hagenbuch & Meier, 2003). Oatp1 is also localized, in addition to the basolateral plasma membrane of hepatocytes, at the apical membranes of kidney proximal tubule (S3 segment). Thus, this transporter could be responsible for reabsorption of organic compounds that are freely filtered, such as estradiol-17β-glucuronide, or important for the secretion of certain organic compounds that are taken up into proximal tubular cells across the basolateral membrane (Gotoh et al., 2002; Obadait et al., 2012). However, it is surprising that BSP, a known substrate for the Oatp1 transport, is normally secreted negligibly by the kidney in non-pathological conditions.

Regulation of Oatp1 expression and function occurs at transcriptional and post-transcriptional levels and is, at least in part, tissue-specific. Thus, while in the kidney Oatp1 expression is stimulated by testosterone and inhibited by estrogens, hepatic Oatp1 expression is not influenced by sex hormones (Gotoh et al., 2002; Wood et al., 2005; Rost et al., 2005). Functional down regulation of Oatp1 has been demonstrated via serine phosphorylation by extracellular ATP (Hagenbuch & Meier, 2004). In addition, protein kinase C activation leads to decreased transport of estrone-3-sulfate in Oatp1 expressing *X. laevis* oocytes (Geier et al., 2007; Planchamp et al, 2007).

In rats with cholestasis due to bile duct ligation, the hepatic expression of Oatp1 is down regulated (Geier et al., 2007). This transporter mediates hepatic uptake of numerous organic anions from the systemic circulation. This observation may also be an adaptive change because BDL rats need to restrict excess uptake of various organic anions into hepatocytes. Renal Oatp1 mediates urinary excretion and re-uptake of organic anions at apical (brush border) membrane. It is worth noting that differential processing and trafficking of this transporter in liver and kidney may have important functional and regulatory consequences.

Our data showed that BDL rats have a higher renal expression of Oatp1 protein at apical membranes despite no change in Oatp1 abundance in kidney homogenates (Brandoni et al., 2009b). These observations suggest an alteration in Oatp1 trafficking that might be caused by an increased recruitment of preformed transporters into the membranes or an inhibition in the internalization of membrane transporters. The results of this study have shown that the kidneys are able to adapt rapidly to obstructive cholestasis because BSP renal elimination had increased nearly 30-fold during the first day after induction of bile duct obstruction. This study has shown evidence that this renal adaptation to cholestasis involves an up regulation of the transport capacity of the proximal tubular organic anion-transporting polypeptide 1, Oatp1. This increase in Oatp1 protein units at the apical membrane of renal cells may be a compensatory mechanism for reducing injury to hepatocytes or renal epithelia from cytotoxic materials that may occur in rats with obstructive cholestasis.

Extrahepatic cholestasis induces a complex series of hormonal changes in kidneys (Sheen et al., 2010), which might influence the regulation of Oatp1. Likely several local and systemic factors are produced at the same time, and the role of such factors in the regulation of channels and transporters, in renal cells, in the presence of BDL is still unknown. Probably, the accumulation of bilirubin, bile acids and other potential toxics existing in this cholestatic model may affect transcriptional regulatory mechanisms (e.g. fetal transcription factor, pregnene X receptor) and post-transcriptional regulations (Cheng et al., 2005).

In summary, we present evidence that cholestasis induced by common BDL in the rat induces a redistribution in renal Oatp1 protein units into apical membranes from renal cells (Brandoni et al., 2009b). Moreover, this likely adaptation to hepatic injury, specifically in biliary components elimination, present in this model might explain, at least in part, the huge increase in BSP renal excretion observed in this experimental model.

2.7 Mrp2

This transporter is a primary-active ATP-dependent pump, identified as multidrug resistance-associated protein 2 (Mrp2) (Klaassen & Aleksunes, 2010; Keppler, 2011). As in hepatocytes, renal proximal tubular cells and jejunal cells also exhibit constitutive expression of Mrp2 at the apical membrane (Schaub et al., 1997).

Mrp2 is involved in the organic anion transport of a wide variety of potentially toxic endo- and xenobiotics incluiding bilirubin, drugs, and carcinogens, e.g. in the form of amphiphilic anionic conjugates. In addition, Mrp2 mediates the transport of BSP-conjugated derivates (Nies & Keppler, 2007; Passamonti et al. 2009). It has also been described that Mrp2 mediates PAH transport in kidneys (Van Aubel et al., 2000; Leier et al., 2000).

In obstructive jaundice, adaptive mechanisms may permit the liver adapts to the higher load of biliary constituents in part by altering the expression of hepatobiliary transporters. In fact, studies of the regulation of the canalicular Mrp2 transporter have described reduced levels of mRNA and protein in rats after bile duct ligation (Denson et al., 2002; Dietrich et al., 2004).

Scarce data is available reporting the role of extrahepatic tissues in Mrp2 substrate disposition under conditions of deficient biliary secretory function. Lee et al. (2001) have reported that the up regulation in Mrp2 protein in kidney occurred as early as one day after BDL. On the other hand, Tanaka et al. (2002) have evaluated renal Mrp2 function by PAH clearance in rats with obstructive jaundice. PAH clearance was significantly increased after BDL. They also found an increased in mRNA and protein expression of Mrp2 in BDL animals. In this work, the effect of conjugated bilirubin, unconjugated bilirubin, human bile, and sulfate-conjugated bile acid on Mrp2 gene expression was also evaluated in human renal proximal tubular epithelial cells. They have described that the mRNA expression of Mrp2 increased in these renal cells after treatment with conjugated bilirubin, sulfate-conjugated bile acid or human bile. These results suggest that increased renal Mrp2 is functionally active during obstructive jaundice and the increased Mrp2 expression in the kidneys may provide an alternative pathway for accelerating excretion of bilirubin conjugates during obstructive jaundice.

It has been demonstrated a minor role of the intestine in compensating for altered liver Mrp2 mediated secretory function. In fact, Dietrich *et al.* (2004) have indicated that the expression of Mrp2 in the intestine was down regulated in rats with obstructive cholestasis. A role for increased levels of interleukin-1β was implicated in down-regulation of Mrp2 in both liver and intestine from rats undergoing extrahepatic cholestasis. It was demonstrated that decreased binding of RARα:RXRα nuclear receptor dimer to the promoter region of Mrp2 in BDL rats, due to increased levels of interleukin-1β, accounts for Mrp2 down-regulation in liver. In contrast, renal cortex exhibits up-regulation of expression and function of Mrp2 in BDL rats, which likely results from preserved levels of RARα:RXRα dimer in this tissue. Additionally, it was shown increased renal tubular conversion of 1-chloro-2,4-dinitrobenzene (CDNB) to its glutathione conjugate dinitrophenyl-S-glutathione (DNP-SG) followed by subsequent Mrp2-mediated secretion into urine that partially compensates for altered liver function in experimental obstructive cholestasis (Villanueva et al., 2006). It is worth noting that these results might also explain the increase in BSP and PAH excreted load seen in BDL rats (Brandoni & Torres, 2009; Brandoni et al., 2010; Brandoni et al., 2003a).

In summary, these results confirm that the up regulation of the apical transporter Mrp2 in kidneys is involved in the higher secretion into urine of organic anions, such as BSP, PAH and DNP-SG. The current data demonstrate the relevance of the renal elimination, particularly under conditions of impaired biliary secretory function, as occurs in obstructive cholestasis that partially compensates for altered liver function in this pathology.

3. Conclusions

The higher expression of Oat1 and BBBP at the basolateral domain of renal tubular cells together with the increased expression of Mrp2 at apical membrane could justify the increased excretion of PAH and FS described after 21 h of obstructive jaundice (Brandoni et al., 2003a; Brandoni et al., 2006; Brandoni et al., 2003b; Brandoni et al., 2004a; Brandoni et al., 2004b; Tanaka et al., 2002; Villanueva et al., 2006).

As it has been already mentioned, BSP is an organic anion mainly excreted by the liver, which is a substrate for several carrier proteins such as Oat3, Oatp1, Mrp2 and bilitranslocase. We have demonstrated an increase in BSP urinary excretion in rats with extrahepatic cholestasis associated with a higher expression of Oatp1 in apical membranes and an unchanged expression of Oat3 in basolateral membranes from kidneys (Brandoni et al, 2003a; Brandoni et al., 2006; Brandoni & Torres, 2009b). Moreover, Mrp2 up regulation in kidneys from BDL rats has been described (Tanaka et al., 2002; Villanueva et al., 2006).

The increase in Oat1, bilitranslocase and BBBP protein units at renal basolateral membrane together with the increased expression of Oatp1 and Mrp2, and the fall in ABST function, at the apical domain of renal cells may be a compensatory mechanism for protecting hepatocytes or kidney cells from cytotoxic substances that accumulate in the presence of obstructive cholestasis. The upregulation observed in BTL, BBBP, Oatp1 and Mrp2 might explain the dramatic increase in BSP renal elimination displayed in this pathology (Brandoni et al., 2009b; Brandoni et al., 2010).

On the other hand, it has also been found that urinary excretion of bile acids is markedly increased in obstructive liver diseases (Ostrow, 1993). The increase in bile acids urinary excretion may be a consequence of the fact that the amount of filtered bile acids in cholestasis exceeds the maximum capacity for tubular reabsorption. But it may also involve adaptive mechanisms of the kidneys, such as a decline of tubular apical reabsorption of bile acids and an enhanced tubular basolateral uptake.

Mrp2 and the sodium-dependent bile salt transporter ABST are two renal apical bile acids carriers; Mrp2 mediates the exit of bile acids from the cells and ABST is involved in their reabsorption. As was previously mentioned, Mrp2 is upregulated (Tanaka et al., 2002) and there is a fall in the function of ABST (Schlattjan et al., 2003) in the presence of acute extrahepatic cholestasis. Both mechanisms may also contribute to the increased excretion of bile acids in the presence of this pathology. On behalf of the basolateral domain, Oat3 transports bile acids from the blood into the cells. As it has been mentioned earlier, its expression at the basolateral membrane does not change in this experimental model of 21 h of acute extrahepatic cholestasis in rats (Brandoni et al., 2006a).

Figure 2 shows a summary of expression modifications in organic anion transporters detected after acute extrahepatic cholestasis and table 1 shows their consequences in urinary excretions of BSP, PAH and FS.

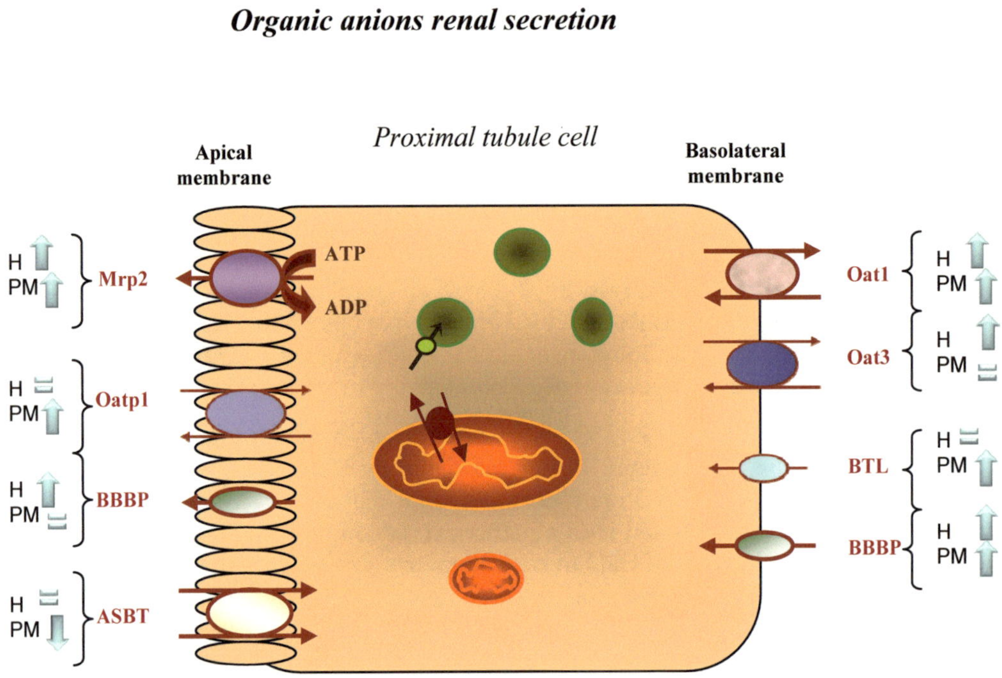

Fig. 2. Expression of the organic anion transporters in proximal renal tubule cell during extrahepatic cholestasis in the rat. For proteins abbreviations see the text. H: homogenate; PM: plasma membrane.

	Renal excreted loads		
Protein abundance	PAH	FS	BSP
Oat1 ↑	↑	↑	
BTL ↑			↑
BBBP[a] ↑	↑		↑
Oatp1 ↑			↑
Mrp2 ↑	↑		↑

([a])Apical expression of BBBP was not changed compared to sham animals while basolateral expression was increased as indicated in the table.

Table 1. Renal organic anions transporters: basolateral and apical membrane proteins in proximal tubule cell. The table summarizes our results about the renal excretion of the organic anions, PAH, FS and BSP and their relationship with renal expression of the organic anion transporters studied in rats after 21 h of BDL.

To sum up, as a consequence of the hepatic function impairment, alterations in the renal elimination of organic anions were observed. The higher abundances of the organic anions carriers detected in rats with extrahepatic cholestasis might explain the higher renal capacity to eliminate distinct negatively charge compounds in this group of rats. These results suggest a relevant role of these transporters in renal elimination of those organic anions excreted mainly by liver, in the presence of the obstructive cholestasis.

The knowledge of how these transporters are regulated in the presence of pathological states, such as extrahepatic cholestasis, will help to design optimal therapeutics regimens for the most correct use of negatively charged organic drugs.

4. Acknowledgment

This study was supported by grants from: Fondo para la Investigación Científica y Tecnológica (FONCYT), Consejo Nacional de Investigaciones Científicas y Técnicas (CONICET), Universidad Nacional de Rosario (UNR). The authors thank to Prof. H. Endou and to Dr N. Anzai (Department of Pharmacology and Toxicology, Kyorin University School of Medicine, Tokyo, Japan) for kindly providing Oat1 and Oat3 specific antibodies, to Prof. S. Passamonti (Department of Life Science, Trieste University, Italy) for kindly providing BTL specific antibodies and to Prof. W. Stremmel (Medizinische Universitatsklinik, Heidelberg University, Germany) for kindly providing BBBP specific antibodies.

5. References

Anzai, N.; Kanai, Y. & Endou, H. (2006). Organic anion transporter family: current knowledge. *J. Pharmacol. Sci.* Vol.100, 411-426.

Bakhiya, A.; Bahn, A.; Burckhardt, G. & Wolff, N. (2003). Human organic anion transporter 3 (hOAT3) can operate as an exchanger and mediate secretory urate flux. *Cell. Physiol. Biochem.* Vol.13, 249-256.

Barnes, S.; Gollan, J.L. & Billing B.H. (1977). The role of tubular reabsorption in the renal excretion of bile acids. *Biochem. J.* Vol.166, 65-73.

Boyer, J.L.; Trauner, M.; Mennone, A.; Soroka, C.J.; Cai, S.Y.; Moustafa, T.; Zollner, G.; Lee, J.Y & Ballatori, N. (2006). Upregulation of a basolateral FXR-dependent bile acid efflux transporter OSTalpha-OSTbeta in cholestasis in humans and rodents. *Am J Physiol Gastrointest* 290: G1124-G1130 .

Brandoni, A.; Quaglia, N.B. & Torres, A.M. (2003a). Compensation increase in organic anion excretion in rats with acute biliary. *Pharmacology* Vol.68, 57-63.

Brandoni, A.; Villar, S.R.; Stremmel, W. & Torres, A.M. (2003b). Proteínas transportadoras involucradas en la eliminación renal de bromosulfoftaleína en ratas con colestasis extrahepática. *Medicina* Vol.63, No.5, 189 (Abstract).

Brandoni, A.; Villar, S.R.; Quaglia, N.B. & Torres, A.M. (2004a). Improvement in renal excretion of different organic anions in rats with extrahepatic cholestasis. *Liver International* Vol.24, No.4, P-63 (Abstract).

Brandoni, A.; Villar, S.R.; Quaglia, N.B. & Torres, A.M. (2004b). Elimination of p-aminohippurate (PAH) and sulfobromophthalein (BSP) in rats with extrahepatic cholestasis (EHC) of 21 hours. A comparative study. *Biocell* Vol.28, No.2, 64 (Abstract).

Brandoni, A.; Villar, S.R.; Picena, J.C.; Anzai, N.; Endou, H. & Torres, A.M. (2006a). Expression of rat renal cortical OAT1 and OAT3 in response to acute biliary obstruction. *Hepatology* Vol.43, 1092-1100.

Brandoni, A.; Anzai, N.; Kanai, Y.; Endou, H. & Torres, A.M. (2006b). Renal elimination of p-aminohippurate (PAH) in response to three days of biliary obstruction in the rat. The role of OAT1 and OAT3. *Biochim. Biophys. Acta* Vol.1762, 673-682.

Brandoni, A.; Villar, S. R.; Anzai, N.; Endou, H. & Torres, A. M. (2006c). Modifications in p-aminohippurate renal transport in rats with acute biliary obstruction. *Physiol. Minireviews* Vol.2, 181 (Abstract).

Brandoni, A. & Torres, A.M. (2009a). Extrahepatic cholestasis model, In: *Experimental Surgical Models in the Laboratory Rat*, A. Rigalli, V. Di Loreto (eds), pp 139–141, CRC Press Taylor and Francis Group, Boca Ratón, USA.

Brandoni, A. & Torres, A.M. (2009b). Characterization of the mechanisms involved in the increased renal elimination of bromosulfophthalein during cholestasis: involvement of Oatp1. *J. Histochem. Cytochem.* Vol.57, 449–456.

Brandoni, A. & Torres, A.M. (2010). Expression and function of renal organic anion transporters (Oats) in health and disease. *Current Topics in Pharmacology* 14: 1-9.

Brandoni, A.; Di Giusto, G.; Franca, R.; Passamonti, S. & Torres, A.M. (2010) Expression of kidney and liver bilitranslocase in response to acute biliary obstruction. *Nephron Physiol.* Vol.114, 35-40.

Burckhardt, G.; Kramer, W.; Kurz, G. & Wilson, F.A. (1987). Photoaffinity labeling studies of the rat renal sodium bile salt cotransport system. *Biochem. Biophys. Res. Commun.* Vol.143, 1018-1023.

Burckhardt G. & Pritchard J.B. (2000). Organic anion and cation antiporters, In: *The Kidney. Physiology and Pathophysiology. Third edition.* D.W. Seldin & G. Giebisch (eds), pp 193-222, LIPPINCOTT WILLIAMS & WILKINS, Philadelphia, USA.

Burckhardt, B.C. & Burckhardt, G. (2003). Transport of organic anions across the basolateral membrane of proximal tubule cells. *Rev. Physiol. Biochem. Pharmacol.* Vol.146, 95-158.

Burckhardt, G. & Burckhardt, B.C. (2011). In vitro and in vivo evidence of the importance of organic anion transporters (OATs) in drug therapy, In: *Drug transporters, Handbook of experimental pharmacology 201.* M.F. Fromm & R.B. Kim (eds), pp 29-104, Springer-Verlag, Berlin, Germany.

Cha, S.H.; Sekine, T.; Fukushima, J.I.; Kanai, Y.; Kobayashi, Y.; Goya, T. & Endou, H. (2001). Identification and characterization of human organic anion transporter 3 expressing predominantly in the kidney. *Mol. Pharmacol.* Vol.59, 1277-1286.

Chen, J.; Terada, T.; Ogasawara, K.; Katsura, T. & Inui, K-I. (2008). Adaptive responses of renal organic anion transporter 3 (OAT3) during cholestasis. *Am. J. Physiol.* Vol.295, F247-F252.

Cheng, X.; Maher, J.; Dieter, M.Z. & Klaassen, C.D. (2005) Regulation of mouse organic anion-transporting polypeptides (oatps) in liver by prototypical microsomal enzyme inducers that activate distinct transcription factor pathways. *Drug Metab. Dispos.* Vol.33, 1276-1282.

Christie, D.M.; Dawson, P.A.; Thevananther, S. & Schneider, B.L. (1996). Comparative analysis of the ontogeny of a sodium-dependent bile acid transporter in rat kidney and ileum. *Am. J. Physiol.* Vol.271, G377-G385.

Denk, G.U.; Soroka, C.J.; Takeyama, Y.; Chen, W.S.; Schuetz, J.D. & Boyer, J.L. (2004). Multidrug resistance-associated protein 4 is up-regulated in liver but down-regulated in kidney in obstructive cholestasis in the rat. *J. Hepatol.* Vol.40, 585-591.

Denson, L.A.; Bohan, A.; Held, M.A. & Boyer, J.L. (2002). Organ-specific alterations in RAR alpha:RXR alpha abundance regulate rat Mrp2 (Abcc2) expression in obstructive cholestasis. *Gastroenterology* Vol.123, 599-607.

Dietrich, C.; Geier, A.; Salein, N.; Lammert, F.; Roeb, E.; Oude Elferink, R.P.; Matern, S. & Gartung, C. (2004). Consequences of bile duct obstruction on intestinal expression and function of multidrug resistance-associated protein 2. *Gastroenterology* Vol.126, 1044-1053.

Donner, M.G.; Schumacher, S.; Warskulat, U.; Heinemann, J. & Häussinger, D. (2007). Obstructive cholestasis induces TNF-a- and IL-1b-mediated periportal downregulation of Bsep and zonal regulation of Ntcp, Oatp1a4, and Oatp1b2. *Am. J. Physiol.* Vol.293, G1134–G1146.

Elías, M.M.; Lunazzi, G.C.; Passamonti, S.; Gazzin, B.; Miccio, M.; Stanta, G.; Sottocasa, G.L. & Tiribelli, C. (1990). Bilitranslocase localization and function in basolateral plasma membrane of renal proximal tubule in rat. *Am. J. Physiol.* Vol.259, F559–F564.

El-Sheikh, A.A.K.; Masereeuw, R. & Russel, F.G.M. (2008). Mechanisms of renal anionic druf transport. *Eur. J. Pharmacol.* Vol.585, 245-255.

Eraly, S.A.; Vallon, V.; Vaughn, D.A.; Gangoiti, J.A.; Richter, K.; Nagle, M.; Monte, J.C.; Rieg, T.; Truong, D.M.; Long, J.M.; Barshop, B.A.; Kaler, G. & Nigam, S.K. (2006). Decreased renal organic anion secretion and plasma accumulation of endogenous organic anions in OAT1 knock-out mice. *J. Biol. Chem.* Vol. 281, 5072-5083.

Geier, A.; Dietrich, C.G.; Trauner, M. & Gartung, C. (2007). Extrahepatic cholestasis downregulates Oatp1 by TNF-alpha signalling without affecting Oatp2 and Oatp4 expression and sodium-independent bile salt uptake in rat liver. *Liver Int.* Vol.27, 1056–1065.

Gotoh, Y.; Kato, Y.; Stieger, B.; Meier, P.J. & Sugiyama Y (2002). Gender difference in the Oatp1-mediated tubular reabsorption of estradiol 17beta-D-glucuronide in rats. *Am. J. Physiol.* Vol.282, E1245–1254.

Hasannejad H., Takeda M., Taki K., Shin H.J., Babu E., Jutabha P., Khamdang S., Aleboyeh M., Onozato M.L., Tojo A., Enomoto A., Anzai N., Narikawa S., Huang X., Niwa T. & Endou H. (2004). Interactions of human organic anion transporters with diuretics. J. *Pharmacol. Exp. Ther.* Vol.308, 1021-1029.

Hirohata, Y.; Fujii, M.; Okabayashi, Y.; Nagashio, Y.; Tashiro, M.; Imoto, I.; Akiyama, T. & Otsuki, M. (2002). Stimulatory effects of bilirubin on amylase release from isolated rat pancreatic acini. *Am. J. Physiol.* Vol.282, 242–256.

Hagenbuch, B. & Meier, P.J. (2003). The superfamily of organic anion transporting polypeptides. *Biochim. Biophys. Acta* Vol.1609, 1–18.

Hagenbuch, B. & Meier, P.J. (2004). Organic anion transporting polypeptides of the OATP/SLC21 family: phylogenetic classification as OATP/ *SLCO* superfamily, new nomenclature and molecular/functional properties. *Pflügers Arch.* Vol.447, 653–65.

Hagenbuch, B. (2010). Drug uptake systems in liver and kidney: a historic perspective. *Clin. Pharmacol. Ther.* 87:39-47.

Kalliokoski, A. & Niemi, M. (2009). Impact of OATP transporters on pharmacokinetics. *Br. J. Pharmacol.* Vol.158, 693-705.

Keppler, D. (2011). Multidrug resistance proteins (MRPs, ABCCs): importance for pathophysiology therapy, In: *Drug transporters, Handbook of experimental pharmacology 201*. M.F. Fromm & R.B. Kim (eds), pp 299-323, Springer-Verlag, Berlin, Germany.

Klaassen, C.D. & Aleksunes, L.M. (2010). Xenobiotic, bile acid, and cholesterol transporters: function and regulation. *Pharmacol. Rev.* Vol.62, 1-96.

Kojima, R.; Sekine, T.; Kawachi, M.; Cha, S.H.; Suzuki, Y. & Endou, H. (2002). Immunolocalization of multispecific organic anion transporters, OAT1, OAT2, and OAT3, in rat kidney. *J. Am. Soc. Nephrol.* Vol.13, 848-857.

Kwak, J.O. ; Kim, H-W. ; Oh, K-J. ; Kim, D.S. ; Han, K.O. & Cha, S.H. (2005). Colocalization and interaction of organic anion transporter 1 with caveolin-2 in the kidney. *Exp. Mol. Med.* Vol.37, 204–212.

Lazaridis, K.N.; Pham, L.; Tietz, P., Marinelli, R.A.; deGroen, P.C.; Levine, S.; Dawson, P.A. & LaRusso, N.F. (1997). Rat cholangiocytes absorb bile acids at their apical domain via the ileal sodium-dependent bile acid transporter. *J. Clin. Invest.* Vol.100, 2714-2721.

Lee, J.; Azzaroli, F.; Wang, L., Soroka, C.J.; Gigliozzi, A.; Setchell, K.D.; Kramer, W. & Boyer, J.L. (2001). Adaptive regulation of bile salt transporters in kidney and liver in obstructive cholestasis in the rat. *Gastroenterology* Vol.121, 1473-1484.

Leier, I.; Hummel-Eisenbeiss, J.; Cui, Y. & Keppler, D. (2000). ATP-dependent paraaminohippurate transport by apical multidrug resistance protein MRP2. *Kidney Int.* Vol.57, 1636–1642.

Nies, A.T. & Keppler, D. (2007). The apical conjugate efflux pump ABCC2 (MRP2). *Pflügers Arch* Vol.453, 643 - 659.

Obaidat, A.; Roth, M. & Hagenbuch, B. (2012). The expression and function of organic anion transporting polypeptides in normal tissues and in cancer. *Annu. Rev. Pharmacol. Toxicol.* Vol.52, 135–51.

Ostrow, J.D. (1993). Metabolism of bile salts in cholestasis in humans, In: *Hepatic Transport and Bile Secretion: Physiology and Pathophysiology*, N. Tavolin, P.D. Berk (eds), pp 673–712, Raven Press, New York, USA.

Planchamp, C.; Hadengue, A.; Stieger, B.; Bourquin, J.; Vonlaufen, A.; Frossard, J-L.; Quadri, R.; Becker, C.D. & Pastor, C.M. (2007). Function of Both Sinusoidal and Canalicular Transporters Controls the Concentration of Organic Anions within Hepatocytes. *Mol. Pharmacol.* Vol.71, 1089-1097.

Passamonti, S.; Terdoslavich, M.; Franca, R.; Vanzo, A.; Tramer, F.; Braidot, E.; Petrussa, E. & Vianello, A. (2009). Bioavailability of flavonoids: a review of their membrane transport and the function of bilitranslocase in animal and plant organisms. *Curr. Drug Metab.* Vol.10, 369–394.

Paumgartner, G.& Beuers, U. (2004). Mechanisms of action and therapeutic efficacy of ursodeoxycholic acid in cholestatic liver disease. *Clin. Liver Dis.* Vol.8, 67-81.

Pei, Q.L.; Kobayashi, Y.; Tanaka, Y.; Taguchi, Y.; Higuchi, K.; Kaito, M.; Ma. N.; Semba, R.; Kamisako, T. & Adachi, Y. (2002). Increased expression of multidrug resistance-associated protein 1 (mrp1) in hepatocyte basolateral membrane and renal tubular epithelia after bile duct ligation in rats. *Hepatol. Res.* Vol.22, 58-64

Plebani, M.; Panozzo, M.P.; Basso, D.; De Paoli, M.; Biasin, R. & Infantolino, D. (1999). Cytokines and the progression of liver damage in experimental bile duct ligation. *Clin. Exp. Pharmacol. Physiol.* Vol. 26, 358-363.

Reichen, J. & Simon, F.R. (1988). Cholestasis, In: *The Liver: Biology and Pathobiology. Second Edition*, I.M. Arias, W.B. Jakoby, H. Popper, D. Schachter & D.A. Shafritz (eds), pp 1105-1124, Raven Press Ltd., New York, USA.

Rizwan, A.N. & Burckhardt, G. (2007). Organic anion transporters of the SLC22 family: biopharmaceutical, physiological, and pathological roles. *Pharm. Res.* Vol.24, 450-470.

Rost, D.; Herrmann, T.; Sauer, P.; Schmidts, H.L.; Stieger, B.; Meier, P.J.; Stremmel, W. & Stiehl, A. (2003). Regulation of rat organic anion transporters in bile salt-induced cholestatic hepatitis: effect of ursodeoxycholate. *Hepatology;* 38: 187-195.

Rost, D.; Kopplow, K.; Gehrke, S.; Mueller, S.; Friess, H.; Ittrich, C.; Mayer, D. & Stiehl, A. (2005). Gender-specific expression of liver organic anion transporters in rat. *Eur. J. Clin. Invest.* Vol.35, 635-643.

Rudman, D. & Kendall, F.E. (1957). Bile acid content of human serum. II. The binding of cholanic acid by human plasma proteins. *J. Clin. Invest.* Vol.36, 538-542.

Russel, F.G.M.; Masereeuw, R. & van Aubel, R.A.M.H. (2002). Molecular aspects of renal anionic drug transport. *Annu. Rev. Physiol.* Vol.64, 563-594.

Schaub, T.P.; Kartenbeck, J.; König, J.; Vogel, O.; Witzgall, R.; Kritz, W. & Keppler, D (1997). Expression of the conjugate export pump encoded by the mrp2 gene in the apical membrane of kidney proximal tubules. *J. Am. Soc. Nephrol.* Vol.8, 1213-1221.

Schlattjan, J.H.; Winter, C. & Greven, J. (2003) Regulation of renal tubular bile acid transport in the early phase of an obstructive cholestasis in the rat. *Nephron Physiol.* Vol.95, 49-56.

Sheen, J-M. , Huang, L-T.; Hsieh, C-S.; Chen, C-C.; Wang, J-Y. & Tain, Y-L. (2010). Bile duct ligation in developing rats: temporal progression of liver, kidney, and brain damage. *J. Pediatr. Surg.* Vol.45, 1650-1658.

Slitt, A.L.; Allen, K.; Morrone, J.; Aleksunes, L.M.; Chen, C.; Maher, J.M.; Manautou, J.E.; Cherrington, N.J. & Klaassen, C.D. (2007). Regulation of transporter expression in mouse liver, kidney, and intestine during extrahepatic cholestasis. *Biochim. Biophys. Acta* Vol.1768, 637-647.

Stremmel, W.; Gerber, M.A.; Glezerov, V.; Thung , S.N.; Kochwa, S. & Berk, P. (1983). Physicochemical and immunohistochemical studies of a sulfobromophthalein and bilirubin-binding protein from rat liver plasma membrane. *J. Clin. Invest.* Vol.71, 1796-1805.

Stremmel, W. & Berk, P. (1986). Hepatocellular uptake of sulfobromophthalein and bilirubin is selectively inhibited by an antibody to the liver plasma membrane sulfobromophthalein/bilirubin binding protein. *J. Clin. Invest.* Vol.78, 822-826.

Sweet, D.H.; Miller, D.S.; Pritchard, J.B.; Fujiwara, Y.; Beier, D.R. & Nigam, S.K. (2002). Impaired organic anion transport in kidney and choroid plexus of organic anion transporter 3 (Oat3 (Slc22a8)) knockout mice. *J. Biol. Chem.* Vol.277, 26934-26943.

Sweet, D.H.; Chan, L.M.; Walden, R.; Yang, X.P.; Miller, D.S. & Pritchard, J.B. (2003). Organic anion transporter 3 (Slc22a8) is a dicarboxylate exchanger indirectly coupled to the Na+ gradient. *Am. J. Physiol.* Vol.284, F763-F769.

Sweet, D.H. (2005). Organic anion transporter (Slc22a) family members as mediators of toxicity. *Toxicol. Appl. Pharmacol.* Vol.204, 198-215.

Tanaka, Y.; Kobayashi, Y.; Gabazza, E.C.; Higuchi, K.; Kamisako, T.; Kuroda, M.; Takeuchi, K.; Iwasa, M.;, Kaito, M. & Adachi Y. (2002)Increased renal expression of bilirubin glucuronide transporters in a rat model of obstructive jaundice. *Am. J. Physiol. Gastrointest.* Vol.282, G656-G662.

Tiribelli, C.; Lunazzi, G.; Luciani, M.; Panfili, E.; Gazzin, B.; Liut, G.; Sandri, G. & Sottocasa, G.L. (1978) Isolation of a sulfobromophthalein-binding protein from hepatocyte plasma membrane. *Biochem. Biophys. Acta* Vol. 531, 105–112.

Tojo A., Sekine T., Nakajima N., Hosoyamada M., Kanai Y., Kimura K. & Endou H. (1999). Immunohistochemical localization of multispecific renal organic anion transporter 1 in rat kidney. *J. Am. Soc. Nephrol.* Vol.10, 464-471.

Torres, A.M.; Lunazzi, G.C.; Stremmel, W. & Tiribelli, C. (1993). Bilitranslocase and sulfobromophthalein/bilirubin-binding protein are both involved in the hepatic uptake of organic anions. *Proc. Natl. Acad. Sci. USA* Vol.90, 8136–8139.

Torres, A.M. (1997). Mechanistic aspects in the hepatic uptake of long chain free fatty acids, bile acids and non-bile acids cholephilic organic anions. *Current Topics in Pharmacology* Vol.3, 137-144.

Torres, A.M.; Anzai, N. & Endou, H. (2008). Renal organic anion transporters: Knowledge from animal models. *Current Topics in Pharmacology* Vol.12, 45-50.

Torres, A.M. (2008). Renal elimination of organic anions in cholestasis. *World Journal of Gastroenterology* 14 (43) 6616-6621, (November 2008) ISSN 1007-9327.

Van Aubel, R.A.M.; Peters, J.G.; Masereeuw, R.; Van Os, C.H. & Russel, F.G.M. (2000). Multidrug resistance protein Mrp2 mediates ATP-dependent transport of classical renal organic anion p-aminohippurate. *Am. J. Physiol.* Vol.279, F713–F717.

Van Wert, A.L.; Gionfriddo, M.R. & Sweet, D.H. (2010). Organic anion transporters: Discovery, Pharmacology, Regulation and Roles in Pathophysiology. *Biopharm. Drug Dispos.* Vol.31, 1-71.

Vanzo, A.;Terdoslavich, M.; Brandoni, A.; Torres, A.M.; Vrhovsek, U.& Passamonti, S. (2008). Uptake of grape anthocyanins into the rat kidney and the involvement of bilitranslocase. *Mol. Nutr. Food Res.* Vol.52, 1106–1116.

Villanueva, S.S.M.; Ruiz, M.L.; Soroka, C.J.; Cai, S.H.; Luquita, M.G.; Torres, A.M.; Sánchez Pozzi, E.J.; Pellegrino, J.M.; Boyer, J.L.; Catania, V.A. & Mottino, A.D. (2006). Hepatic and extrahepatic synthesis and disposition of dinitrophenyl-Sglutathione in bile duct-ligated rats. *Drug Metab. Dispos.* Vol.34, 1301–1309.

Weiner, I.M.; Glasser, J.E. & Lack, L. (1964). Renal excretion of bile acids: Taurocholic, glycocholic and cholic acids. *Am. J. Physiol.* Vol.2076, 964-970.

Wilson, F.A.; Burckhardt, G.; Murer, H.; Rumrich, G. & Ullrich, K.J. (1981). Sodium-coupled taurocholate transport in the proximal convolution of the rat kidney in vivo and in vitro. *J. Clin. Invest.* Vol.67, 1141-1150.

Wood, M.; Ananthanarayanan, M.; Jones, B. ; Wooton-Kee, R.; Hoffman, T.; Suchy, F.J. & Vore M. (2005). Hormonal Regulation of Hepatic Organic Anion Transporting Polypeptides. *Mol. Pharmacol.* Vol.68, 218-225.

Wright, S.H. & Dantzler, W.H. (2004). Molecular and cellular physiology of renal organic cation and anion transport. *Physiol. Rev.* Vol.84, 987-1049.

Part 2

Experimental Models of Cholestasis

4

Drug-Induced Models of Cholestasis and Lysosomes

T.A. Korolenko, O.A. Levina, E.E. Filjushina and N.G. Savchenko
Institute of Physiology, Siberian Branch of Russian Academy of Medical Sciences,
Novosibirsk
Russia

1. Introduction

Cholestasis, caused by the interrupted excretion of bile, resulting in an accumulation of bile products in the body fluids is characteristic of many human liver diseases (Sherlock & Dooley, 1997). Experimental animal models of cholestasis allow the understanding of pathophysiological mechanisms involved and their clinical correlates (Chang et al., 2005; Chandra & Brower, 2004). The most common experimental models of intrahepatic cholestasis are estrogen-induced, endotoxin-induced and drug-induced cholestasis (Rodriguez-Garay, 2003). Drug-induced cholestasis was described during treatment by different drugs in medical clinic and in experimental research. In experimental medicine, α-naphthylisothiocyanate (ANIT) treatment has been extensively used, permitting to describe not only cholestatic alterations but also compensatory mechanisms. The animal model and transport protein studies are necessary for the progressive understanding of congenital and acquired human cholestasis, and regulatory mechanisms which operate on liver cells. Continuous bile formation is an important function of the liver, and bile is used as a vehicle for the secretion of bile acids and the excretion of lipophilic endo- and xenobiotics (Meier and Stieger, 2000; Hsien et al., 2006). Molecular and cellular mechanisms of intrahepatic cholestasis development are important for understanding of role of different factors in this process and effective therapy. Lysosomes are connected with bile secretion, however their role in cholestasis development is still not clear. Human bile revealed high activity of lysosomal enzymes (β-galactosidase, β-N-acetylglucosaminidase, acid phosphatase) which are suggested to be secreted from lysosomes localized in peribiliar zone of hepatocytes (Korolenko et al., 2007). We tested the hypothesis that impaired lysosomal secretion is related to cholestasis development. Earlier in some works it was shown that in mice and rats increased activity of lysosomal enzymes in bile was connected with their increased secretion.

The aim: to study the mechanism of intrahepatic cholestasis development and the role of lysosomes in bile secretion and cholestasis development. The following models of experimental cholestasis have been used and analyzed in our study: known model of intrahepatic cholestasis induced by α–naphtylisothyocyanate (ANIT) and lysosomotropic agent Triton WR 1339.

2. Drugs induced cholestasis and lysosomotropic agents

In inflammatory disorders such as sepsis, bacterial infections, viral hepatitis as well as toxic or drug-induced hepatitis, inflammatory cytokines can impair bile secretion (Jansen & Sturm, 2003; Paumgartner, 2006). Intrahepatic cholestasis of different pathomechanisms was shown to develop during treatment by several medical drugs (Krell et al., 1987), some of them possessed by lysosomotropic action. According to concept of de Duve et al. (1974) lysosomotropic agents are selectively taken up into lysosomes following their administration to man and animals (Schneider et al., 1997). The effects of lysosomotropic drugs studied *in vivo* and *in vitro* can be used as models of lysosomal storage diseases. These agents include many drugs still used in clinical medicine: aminoglycoside antibiotics, flouroquin antimicrobial agents (ciprofloxacin), amoxicillin/clavulanic acid, phenothiazine derivatives, antiparasitic and anti-inflammatory drugs (chloroquine and suramin, gold sodium thiomalate) and cardiotonic drugs like sulmazol (Schneider et al., 1997). Side-effects to these drugs can be caused partially by their lysosomotropic properties. In addition to drugs, other compounds to which man and animals are exposed (e.g., heavy metals, iron compounds, lantan and gadolinium salts, some cytostatics) are also lysosomotropic. Liver cells, especially Kupffer cells, are known to accumulate lysosomotropic agents. We present our studies which evaluate lysosomal changes in the liver following administration of lysosomotropic agents in experimental animals, and relate them to toxic side-effects or pharmacological action, as was suggested earlier (de Duve et al., 1974). Common features of lysosomal changes include the overload of liver lysosomes by non-digestible material; increased size and number of liver lysosomes; inhibition of several lysosomal enzymes; secondary increase in the activity of some lysosomal enzymes; increased autophagy, and fusion disturbances.

2.1 Biochemical component of bile of intact CBA/C57BL mice

2.1.1 Experimental animals and methods used

All animal procedures were carried out in accordance to approved protocol and recommendations for proper use and care of laboratory animals (European Communities Council Directive 86/609/CEE). Experiments were performed on male CBA/C57BL/6 mice weighting 25-30 g (Institute of Physiology, Siberian Branch of Russian Academy of Medical Sciences, Novosibirsk). To reproduce the model of intrahepatic cholestasis corn oil solution of ANIT was injected intraperitoneally in a single dose of 200 mg/kg (0.2 ml per mouse) (Kodali et al., 2006). The animals were euthanized 24 h after ANIT injection. Triton WR 1339 (Ruger Chemical Co, USA) was dissolved in physiological saline solution and injected intraperitoneally in a single dose of 500 and 1000 mg/kg. The mice were decapitated 24 and 72 h after Triton WR 1339 administration (when significant accumulation of detergent occurred inside of lysosomes). Oil solution of hepatotoxin carbon tetrachloride (CCl_4, 50 mg/kg) was administered intraperitoneally, as a single injection. The mice were used in experiment 24, 48 and 72 h after CCl_4 intoxication. The separate group of animals received Triton WR 1339 two hours before administration of CCl4 in a dose indicated (combined treatment). The mice were deprived of food (15 h before decapitation), but received water *ad libidum*. Blood serum was obtained by centrifugation of samples at 3000 g, +4° C for 20 minutes, using Eppendorf 5415 R centrifuge (Germany). The bile was taken from gall bladder using a microsyringe; the bile samples from 5 mice were combined to measure the lysosomal enzyme activity.

Serum and bile alanine transaminase (ALT) activity (serum marker of hepatocyte cytolisis) was measured with help of commercial Lachema Diagnostica kits (Czech Republic). Activity of alkaline phosphatase and γ-glutamyltransferase (GGTP) were measured using Vital Diagnostics kits (Saint Petersburg, Russia). The increase of serum activity of alkaline phosphatase and GGTP reflects the development of intrahepatic cholestasis in mice. Fluorescent methods were used to measure the following lysosomal enzyme activity: β-D-galactosidase (high specific activity in hepatocytes) in the bile and serum using 4-methylumbellipheryl-β-D-galactopyranoside as a substrate (Melford Laboratories Ltd, Suffolk, UK); β-hexosaminidase or β-N-acetylglucosaminidase (4-MUF-2-acetamido-2-deoxy-β-D-glucopyranoside, Melford Laboratories Ltd. Suffolk, UK) and chitotriosidase - 4-MUF-β-D-N,N', N''-triacetylchitotrioside (Sigma). Fluorescence of samples was measured on Perkin Elmer 650-10S spectrofluorometer at the exitation and emission wavelengths of 360 and 445 nm, respectively. The results were expressed in μmol methylumbelliferone released per liter in min. The data obtained were analyzed statistically, using Student t-test; the differences between the means were significant at $p< 0.05$.

Electron microscopic study of liver cells was provided according to method described by Trout and Viles (1979).

2.1.2 Composition of bile and serum of intact mice

In bile of intact CBA/C57BL mice comparatively to serum the total protein was significantly decreased (more than 60-times), as well as albumin concentration (Table 1); alkaline phosphatase activity in bile is significantly lower as in serum, whereas similar level of ALT activity was noted; AST activity in bile was reduced about twice comparatively to serum of the same animals (Table 1). Activity of lysosomal enzyme β-D-galactosidase was similar in serum and bile of mice (Table 1). One can conclude that murine bile possessed relatively high activity of lysosomal enzyme as well as ALT and AST activity.

Index	Serum	Bile
Total protein, g/L	65.8 ± 2.96	1.140 ± 0.006
Albumin, g/L	30.4 ± 0.70	0.530 ± 0.005
ALT activity, U/L	57.2 ± 1.67	45.4 ± 1.00
AST activity, U/L	201.0 ± 10.60	113.6 ± 14.80
Alkaline phosphatase activity, U/L	268.0 ± 8.16	48.0 ± 6.00
β-D-galactosidase activity, μmol MUF/L per h	12.30 ± 1.33	15.6 ± 0.36

Table 1. Concentration of total protein, albumin and activity of enzymes in serum and bile of Intact CBA/C57BL/6 mice

2.2 ANIT as a model of intrahepatic cholestasis

Experimental models of cholestasis in laboratory animals allow us to evaluate the pathophysiological and molecular mechanisms of this disorder. Some similarities were revealed between experimental cholestasis in animals and cholestasis in patients (Moritoki et al., 2006; Dold et al., 2009). Experimental cholestasis in rats and more rarely in mice can be induced by not only common bile duct ligation, but also by treatment with estrogens, endotoxins, and various medical products. Intrahepatic cholestasis induced by ANIT is a convenient model for studies of hepatocyte injury and compensatory mechanisms in spontaneous recovery of liver function. Changes in hepatocyte transport proteins and dysregulation of bile secretion were revealed in mice with experimental cholestasis (Hsien et al., 2006). Cholestasis in mice and rats was observed in the early period after ANIT treatment (4-8 h), reaching maximum 24 and 48 h after ANIT administration. The severity of cholestasis depended on the dose of ANIT, route and regimen of treatment, and basal level of cytokines (tumor necrosis factor-α, TNF-α). Repeated administration of ANIT to mice is accompanied by the development of biliary cirrhosis; the mechanism of this phenomenon remains unclear (Ferreira et al, 2003).

ANIT is a known hepatotoxic agent that causes acute cholestatic hepatitis with infiltration of neutrophils around bile ducts and necrotic hepatocytes (Kodali et al., 2006; Luyendyk et al., 2011). In this work lysosomal enzyme activity in the bile and blood serum was compared in mice with known experimental intrahepatic cholestasis model induced by ANIT and by lysosomotropic agent Triton WR 1339. ANIT (Aldrich, USA) was administered to mice as an oil solution i.p., single, in a dose of 200 mg/kg. The increase in the concentration of total bilirubin (86.2±8.6 *versus* 9.9±0.8 mmol/L in the control, $p<0.001$) and conjugated bilirubin (45.6±4.3 *versus* 6.10±0.39 mmol/L in the control, $p<0.001$) in blood serum reflected the development of cholestasis in mice. The development of intrahepatic cholestasis was confirmed by the increase in activity of alkaline phosphatase and γ-glutamyltransferase (GGTP) in blood serum. β-Galactosidase, β-hexosaminidase and chitotriosidase activity significantly increased in the bile, but decreased in the serum of mice after treatment with ANIT (Table 2). Our results indicate that intrahepatic cholestasis is manifested in increased secretion of lysosomal glycosidases into the bile. It was suggested that bile components can aggravate damage to liver cells by affecting the processes of hepatocyte apoptosis and necrosis. ANIT dramatically increased serum GGTP activity (Figure 1), indicating severe cholestasis development according to ALT and AST (Figure 3); there was no change of urine creatinine and uroprotein concentrations (Figure 2). Our results indicate that hepatocyte injury and cholestasis are observed 24 h after ANIT treatment. Total cholesterol concentration increased in blood serum (Figure 4A). Triglyceride level increased, while cholesterol concentration decreased in the bile (Figure 4B). Cholesterol serves as a common precursor of bile acids. The ANIT-induced increase in serum cholesterol concentration reflects lipid metabolism disorder, which is manifested in lipid infiltration of the liver and cholestasis.

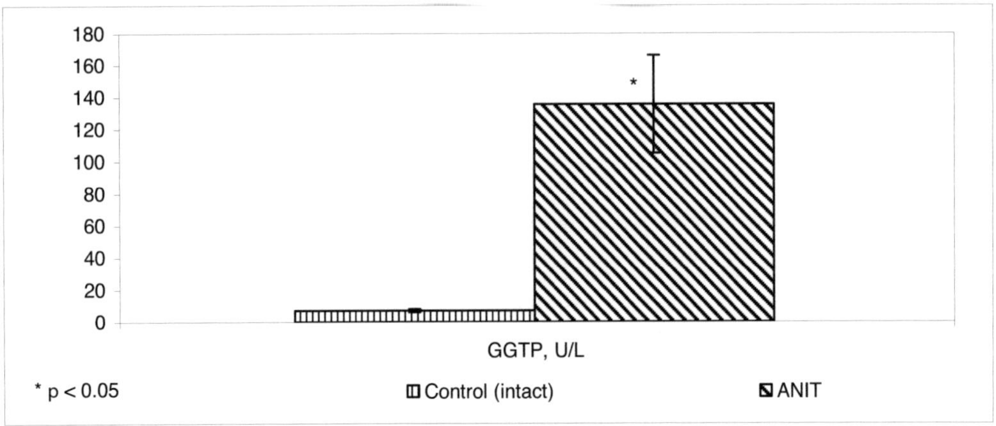

Fig. 1. Effect of ANIT on serum GGTP activity in mice

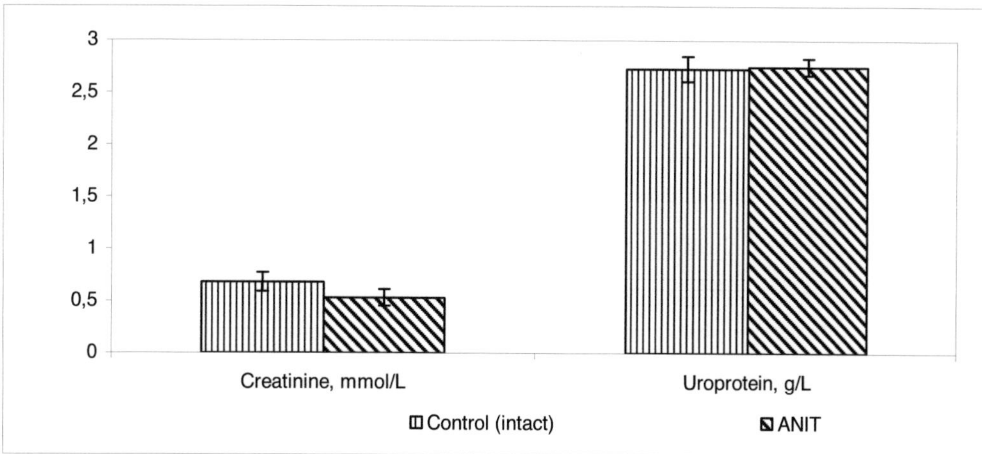

Fig. 2. Effect of ANIT on concentration of creatinine and uroprotein in urine of mice

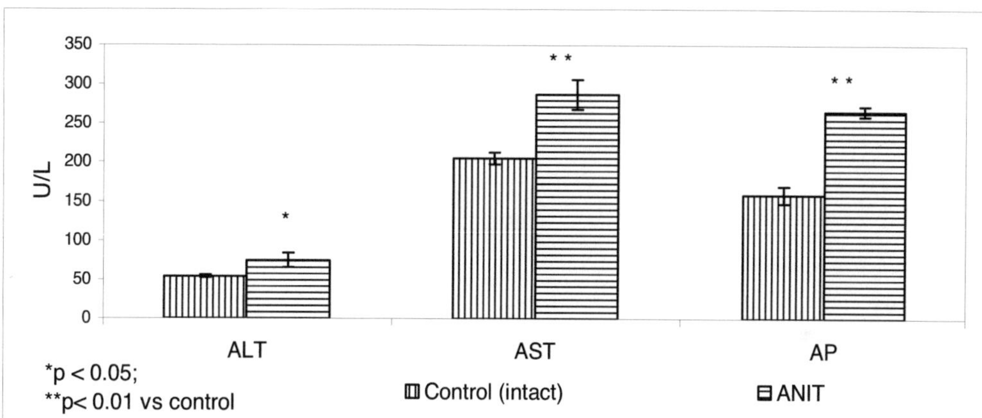

Fig. 3. Effect of ANIT administration in mice on serum ALT, AST and alkaline phosphatase activity

2.2.1 Electron microscopic study of liver (ANIT)

In situ, the increase of gall bladder size of mice was shown (10 μL bile versus 5 μL in intact animals); the color of bile was bright yellow. In general, significant ultrastructural changes in liver cells and microcirculatory region were noted. There was heterogeneity among hepatocyte injury: cells with normal ultrastructure and hepatocytes revealing dystrophic changes were observed. Sinusoids were enlarged, the sinusoidal surface of cells was smooth and revealed only small amount of microvilli. The secretory cell function connected with bile formation was suppressed. The significant dilatation of bile capillaries (Figure 5, 6) was observed, the bile duct had increased oval shape; numerous membraneus material was often noted inside of bile ducts. These electron microscopic data confirmed intrahepatic cholestasis development. In general, liver cell damage included the enlargement of sinusoids and intercellular spaces; enlargement of bile ducts; suppression of protein synthesis in hepatocytes and their dystrophic changes.

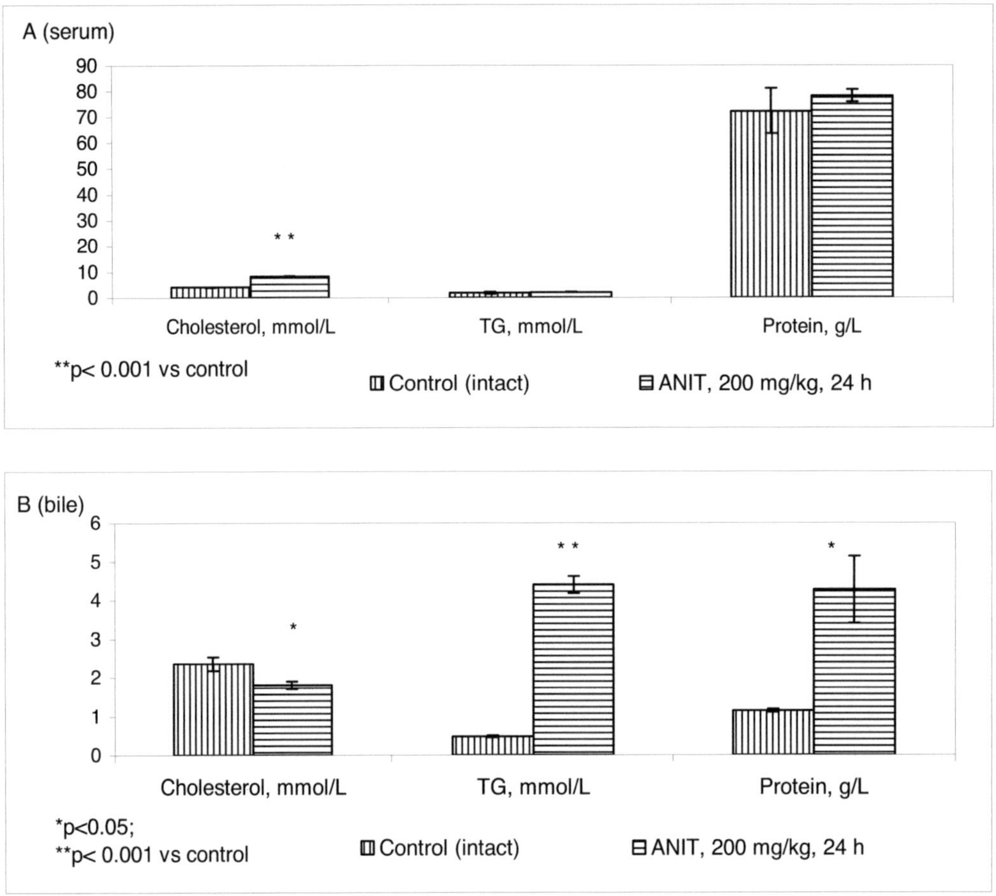

Fig. 4. Concentration of cholesterol, TG and total protein in serum (A) and bile (B) of mice with ANIT administration

2.3 Triton WR 1339t and cholestasis

2.3.1 Triton WR 1339 as a lysosomotropic drug

Triton WR 1339 is non-ionic detergent widely used for isolation of lysosomes (triton-filled lysosomes, tritosomes) in cellular biochemistry (de Duve et al., 1974; Trout and Viles, 1979). Earlier Triton WR 1339 (Tyloxapol) shortly used as a medical drug for treatment of bronchitis. *In vivo* in the doses of 300-1000 mg/kg Triton WR 1339 is taken up by liver cells (mainly by macrophages) and accumulated inside of lysosomes during long period, up to 60 days after the single administration to rats and mice (Schneider et al., 1997). Simultaneously, Triton WR 1339 was shown to induce significant hypercholesterolemia and, especially, hypertriglyceridemia in rats and mice and other laboratory animals, in a dose-dependent manner (Abe et al., 2007; Korolenko et al., 2011). Triton WR 1339 administration to mice (500 mg/kg) was shown to induce significant lipemia sharply increasing both the total lipoprotein-cholesterol and total lipoprotein-triglyceride concentrations in serum of mice. However, the increase in total lipoprotein-triglycerides was much more dramatic (about

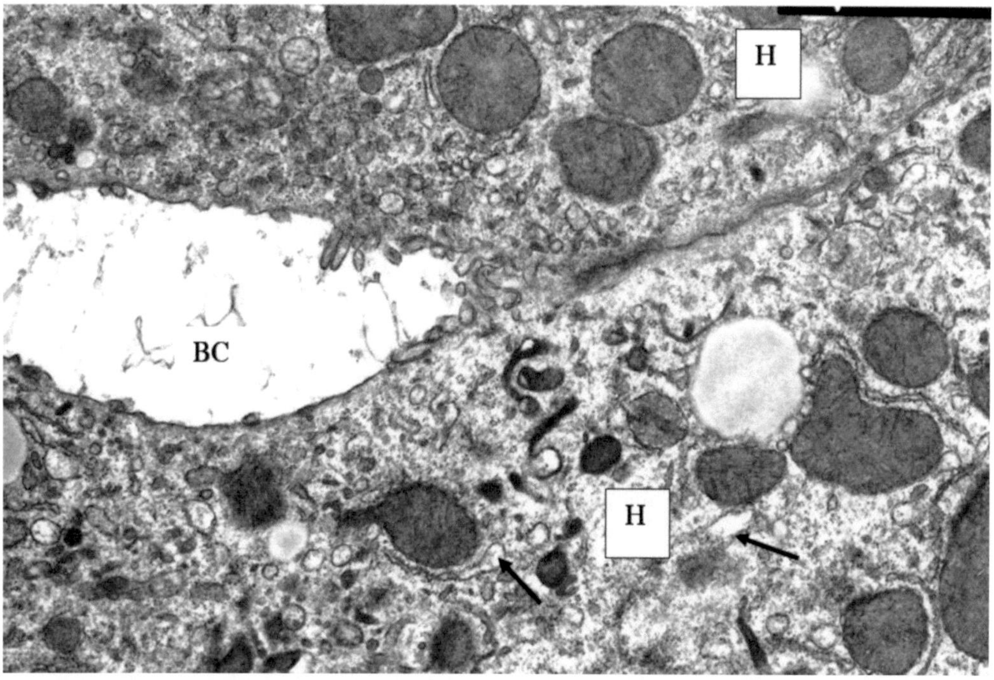

Fig. 5. Hepatocytes of mice with ANIT administration. Enlarged bile capillary (BC), hepatocytes (H) contains enlarged cisterns of endoplasmic reticulum (arrows). X 20 000.

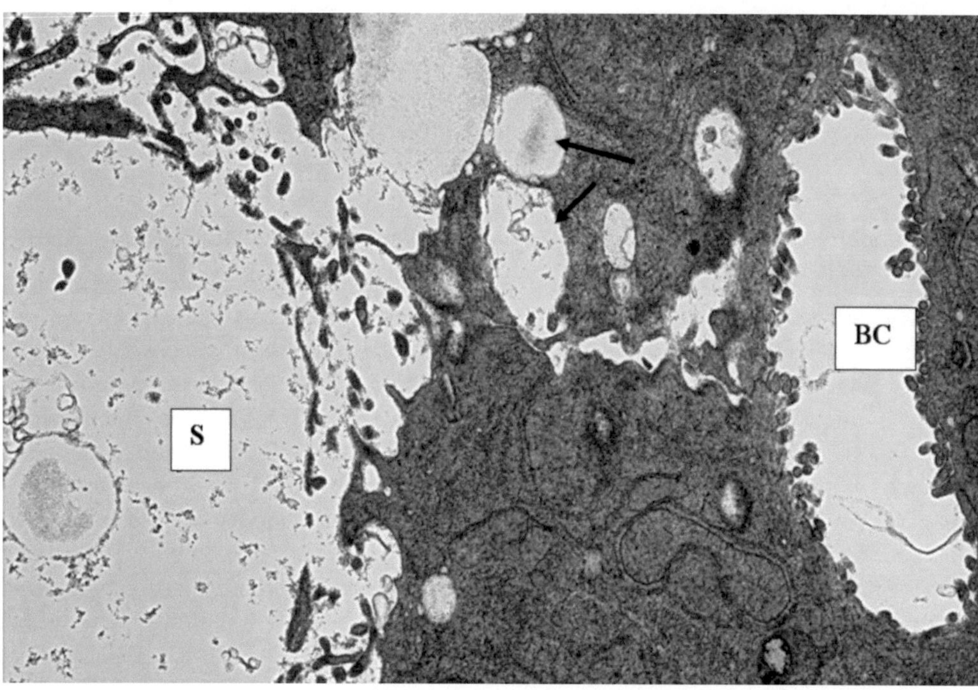

Fig. 6. Electronogram of liver of mice with ANIT administration. Enlarged sinusoid (S) and enlarged bile capillary (BC), hepatocytes contains large vacuoles (arrows). X 20 000.

10-times) than the elevation of the total lipoprotein-cholesterol (about 5-times), relative to control (intact) mice (Korolenko et al., 2011). The Triton WR 1339 hyperlipidemic mouse model is a widely used model for inhibition of lysosomal lipolysis and evaluation of different hypolipidemic drugs (Abe et al., 2007). It was shown that accumulation of Triton WR 1339 occurred simultaneously with some serum lipoproteins inside of liver lysosomes. Triton WR 1339 administration to mice and rats was shown to increase cholesterol synthesis (fatty acids precursor) in liver cells. Possibly, significant hypercholesterolemia induced by Triton WR 1339 administration to mice was related to cholestasis development (presented below), which is not known enough in literature.

2.3.2 Biochemical characteristic of Triton WR 1339-induced cholestasis in mice

Triton WR 1339 (Ruger Chemical Co., USA) was administered in mice as a single injection, i.p., in a dose of 100 mg/100 g, the appropriate animals received the same volume of saline solution. Mice were decapitated 24, 48, 72 h after the single injection. CBA/C57BL/6 male mice of weight 26.8 ± 0.40 g were used. Single administration of Triton WR 1339 (500 mg/kg) in mice was followed by significant increase in concentrations of total cholesterol, TG in serum without changes of the total protein concentration (Figure 7 A). In bile, on the contrary there were no changes of cholesterol and TG level (Figure 7 B); the increase of the total protein concentration was noted in bile.

In mice treated by Triton WR 1339 (500 mg/kg) intrahepatic cholestasis development was confirmed by increased level of serum alkaline phosphatase and GGTP activity (Figure 8). The size of gall-bladder *in situ* was increased, the bile had yellow color. According to electron microscopy study of liver cells numerous triton-filled lysosomes were observed in non-parenchymal (especially in Kupffer cells) and parenchymal cells (Figure 9, 10); enlargement of bile ducts was noted as well as other morphological signs of intrahepatic cholestasis. However, in general the enlargement of bile ducts was shown in a less degree as compare to ANIT-induced model of cholestasis.

2.3.3 The comparison of serum and bile lysosomal enzymes in Triton WR- and ANIT-induced models of cholestasis

The following lysosomal enzymes were compared in two cholestasis models studied: β-D-galactosidase, β-hexosaminidase and chitotriosidase. In intact mice we observed similar activity of β-D-galactosidase in serum and bile, whereas activity of β-hexosaminidase was significantly higher in serum (about 40-times) as compare to bile, as well as chitotriosidase activity (about 6-times higher in serum comparatively to bile) (Table 2). Both models of cholestasis were characterized by decreased β-D-galactosidase and β-hexosaminidase activity in serum (Table 2). However, serum chitotriosidase activity increased in ANIT model and decreased in Triton WR 1339-induced cholestasis (Table 2). In bile all lysosomal enzymes studied - β-D-galactosidase, β-hexosaminidase and chitotriosidase activity were significantly increased (Table 2), especially β-D-galactosidase (about 10-times higher in bile as compare to serum in Triton WR 1339-treated mice (Table 2). In ANIT model we observed higher chitotriosidase activity in bile as compare to Triton WR 1339.

So, both models studied were characterized by increased level of lysosomal enzymes in bile.

Group/Index	Serum	Bile
Intact (β-D-galactosidase, MUF/L per h)	12.3 ± 1.33	12.30 ± 1.63
Triton WR 1339 (β-D-galactosidase, , MUF/L per h)	6.1 ± 0.60 *	117.3 ± 1.40*
ANIT (β-D-galactosidase, , MUF/L per h)	4.6 ± 0.32*	22.2 ± 0.34*
Intact (β-hexosaminidase, μmol MUF/L per min)	7.9 ± 0.95	0.54 ± 0.07
Triton WR 1339 (β-hexosaminidase, μmol MUF/L per min)	4.0 ± 0.47*	2.5 ± 0.20*
ANIT (β-hexosaminidase, μmol MUF/L per min)	1.52 ± 0.05*	1.57 ± 0.10*
Intact (chitotriosidase, μmol MUF/L per min)	20.50 ± 2.79	3.40 ± 0.28
Triton WR 1339 (chitotriosidase, μmol MUF/L per min)	8.90 ± 0.81*	11.85 ± 0.40*
ANIT (chitotriosidase, μmol MUF/L per min)	35.0 ± 2.79*	17.50 ± 3.56*

Table 2. Effect of Triton WR 1339 and ANIT on activity of lysosomal enzymes in serum and bile of mice

*p < 0.01 vs control (intact mice)

Triton WR 1339, 1000 mg/kg, 72 h. ANIT, 200 mg/kg, 24 h. MUF- methylumbelliferyl.

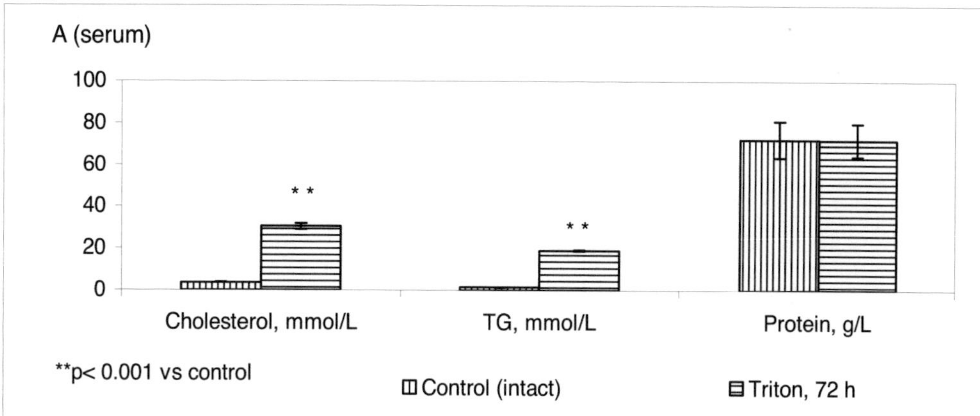

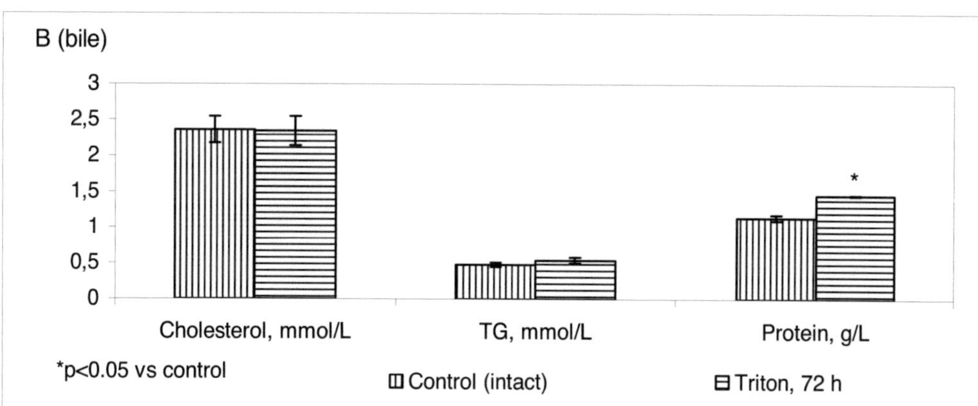

Fig. 7. Effect of Triton WR 1339 administration in mice on serum (A) and bile (B) cholesterol, TG and total protein concentration

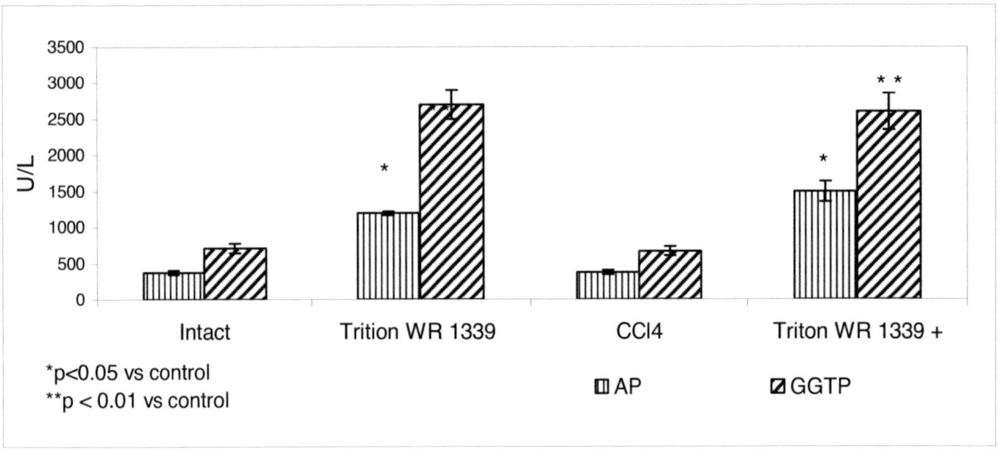

Fig. 8. Effect of Triton WR 1339 on serum alkaline phosphatase (AP) and GGTP activity in intact mice and with acute toxic hepatitis

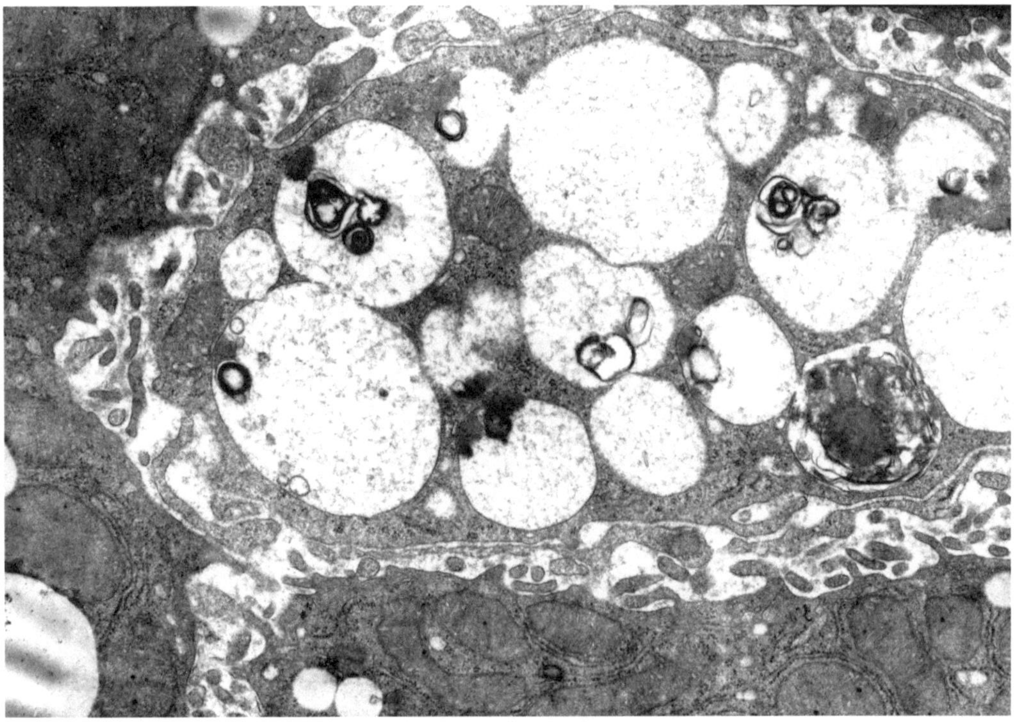

Fig. 9. Electronogram of liver macrophage, triton-filled lysosomes. Triton WR 1339, 1000 mg/kg, 72 h. X 20 000.

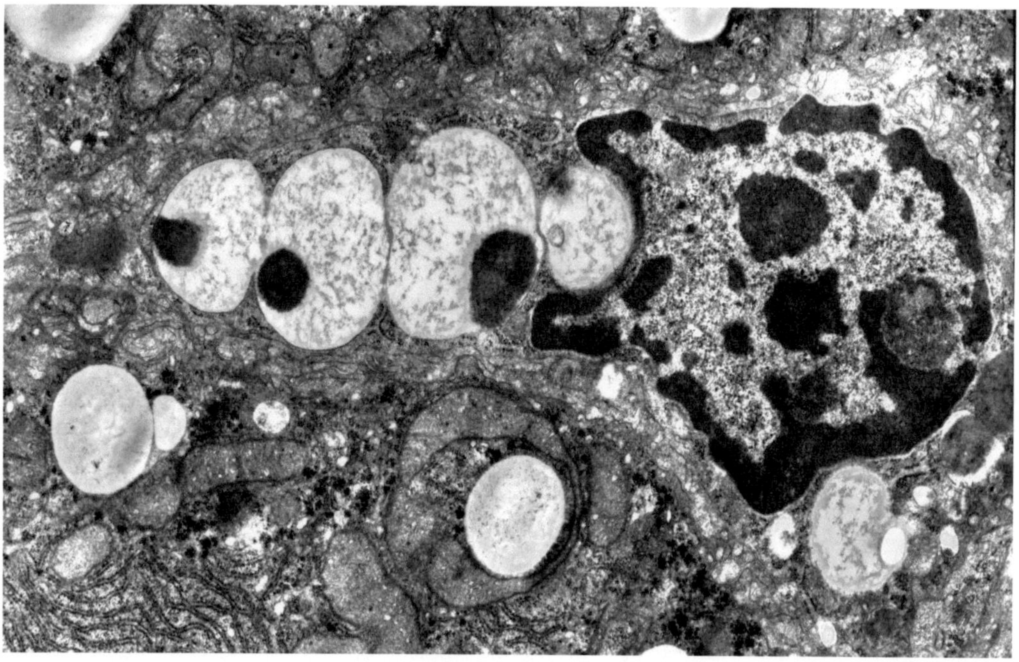

Fig. 10. Electronogram of liver macrophage, Triton WR 1339, 1000 mg/kg, 48 h; enlarged macrophage with numerous triton-filled lysosomes. X 20 000

2.4 Effect of Triton WR 1339 on liver cells ultrastructure

Macroscopically, *in situ;* bile color was bright yellow. The morphological changes of liver cells under Triton WR 1339 administration in rats and mice were described earlier (Trout & Viles, 1979; Schneider et al., 1997), however there was no data collected about the intrahepatic cholestasis development. As was shown before, we observed numerous triton-filled lysosomes in Kupffer cells and also in hepatocytes (Figure 9, 10). The ultrastructural signs of cholestasis induced by Triton WR 1339 in mice included enlargement of bile duct, however these changes were expressed in a lesser degree as compare to ANIT model.

3. The role of liver macrophage in cholestasis development

3.1 Macrophage depression model

Gadolinium chloride is widely used for modeling selective depression of liver macrophages. Selective elimination of the subpopulation of large Kupffer cells, inhibition of receptor-mediated endocytosis and phagocytosis of carbon particles in liver macrophages, increase in the number of mRNA transcripts, and stimulation of TNF-α, IL-1, and IL-6 production were observed 24-48 h after intravenous injection of gadolinium chloride (Ding et al., 2003). The phagocytic function of macrophages recovered and population of liver macrophages was restored after 3 and 4 days, respectively. It was hypothesized that the mechanism of gadolinium accumulation in lysosomes is similar to that for other lysosomotropic agents. This accumulation is accompanied by labilization of lysosomes and leads to cell damage. The consequences of intracellular gadolinium accumulation and its effect on lysosomal functions remain unclear. We studied the kinetics of gadolinium accumulation in the liver and its effects on liver lysosomes and activity of lysosomal enzymes in blood serum. Among lysosomal enzymes we have chosen β-N-acetylhexosaminidase, a marker enzyme of liver macrophages, β-D-glucuronidase and β-D-galactosidase, easily solubilized matrix lysosomal enzymes, whose activity varies more significantly in comparison with membrane-bound enzymes. The suppression of functional activity of Kupffer cells was also followed by the changes in activity of blood serum chitotriosidase, a novel macrophage enzyme (Korolenko et al, 2008).

We have shown that accumulation of gadolinium (as lysosomotropic agent) occurred during the period of its maximum uptake (the day 1 after gadolinium chloride *in vivo* injection) followed by decrease of its concentration (days 5-37). Accumulation of gadolinium inside of lysosomes of liver cells led to structural and functional changes in liver lysosomes. Macrophage depression of the affected macrophages was accompanied by a decrease in osmotic fragility of lysosomes on the day 2 and increase in their osmotic susceptibility during repopulation of macrophages on days 5 and 8. The hypotonic treatment of liver homogenates (0.125 M sucrose at 0° C during 30 min) revealed increased free activity of acid phosphatase (as a result of the increased number of secondary lysosomes in the whole polulation of lysosomes).

Macrophage depression induced by gadolinium chloride *in vivo* was used in studies of the role of macrophages in different experimental models. In our study, electron microscopy of liver cells showed that injection of gadolinium chloride (14 mg/kg) in intact mice was followed by a significant decrease in the numerical density (788.0±69.1 *vs.* 1053.0±60.5 per mm^2 in the control, $p<0.01$) and diminished size of liver macrophages. The relative volume of primary lysosomes and, especially of secondary lysosomes was significantly lower than in the control (1.70 ± 0.64 versus 7.60 ± 1.08% in the control, $p<0.01$). High concentration of gadolinium in the liver was associated mainly with selective intralysosomal accumulation of gadolinium in nonparenchymal liver cells (85% of the administered dose, 1 h after gadolinium chloride administration). Liver function tests (measured according to serum ALT activity) remained unchanged under these conditions. The decrease in the number of liver macrophages and lysosomes in these cells was accompanied by a decrease in specific activity of lysosomal enzymes - cathepsin D and cathepsin B in liver homogenates. No changes were found in activities of cathepsin S, a macrophage-specific cysteine protease (Table 3). In serum the total MMP-2 concentration (proenzyme and active enzyme) was also decreased; TIMP-1 concentration (major endogenous MMP inhibitor) remained unchanged in serum (Table 3). These changes were probably related to interaction between Kupffer cells and stellate cells in the liver, which serve as the main source of MMP and TIMP-1. Our results showed that single injection of gadolinium chloride was followed by a decrease in activities of lysosomal cysteine (cathepsin B) and aspartyl proteases (cathepsin D) studied (Table 3). The observed changes were possibly associated with a decrease in the number and functional activity of Kupffer cells.

We studied the role of selective suppression of liver Kupffer cells (induced by gadolinium chloride, in a dose of 14 mg/kg, intravenously) in the development of intrahepatic cholestasis in CBA/C57BL/6 mice (intraperitoneal injection of ANIT in a single dose of 200 mg/kg).

Index	Control (intact mice)	Gadolinium chloride, 14 mg/kg, 24 h
ALT activity in serum, U/L	54.20 ± 1.55	44.6± 6.10
Cathepsin B activity (liver)	0.27 ± 0.02	0.20 ± 0.02*
Cathepsin L activity (liver)	0.46 ± 0.05	0.46 ± 0.03
Cathepsin S activity (liver)	0.030 ± 0.002	0.030 ± 0.001
Cathepsin D activity (liver)	0.10 ± 0.08	0.060± 0.007*
Total MMP-2 concentration in serum, ng/mL	201.5± 4.66	181.70± 4.64*
Serum TIMP-1 concentration, pg/mL	8000.0 ± 1443.4	8450.0 ± 1472.2

Table 3. Effect of gadolinium chloride on activity of lysosomal enzymes in liver and serum concentrations of MMP-2 and TIMP-1 in mice (M ± m)

Note: * $p<0.05$ vs control. Activity of cathepsin B (against fluorogenic substrate Z-Arg-Arg-MCA), cathepsin L (substrate Z-Phe-Arg-MCA), cathepsin S (substrate Z-Val-Val-Arg- MCA, Sigma–Aldrich, USA) in liver homogenates expressed in nmol MCA/min per mg of protein. Cathepsin D activity is espressed in arbitrary units (A_{366}/min per g of protein). MMP-2 and TIMP-1 concentration was measured using commercial ELISA R&D kits. * $p < 0.05$ as compared to intact animals

In the separate experiment it was shown that preliminary administration of gadolinium chloride to ANIT-treated animals was followed by an increase in activities of ALT (133.5±37.6 *vs.* 74.70±9.18 U/L in the ANIT group, p=0.005), alkaline phosphatase (269.1±9.1 *vs.* 158.6±11.1 U/L in the ANIT group, p=0.0001), and γ-glutamyl transpeptidase in urine samples (243.0±10.0 *vs.* 135.8±30.7 U/L in the ANIT group, p<0.05). Hence, the severity of cholestasis and hepatocyte injury increased after combined treatment with gadolinium chloride and ANIT. Aggravation of cholestasis under macrophage suppression in ANIT-treated animals, probably, was associated with the increased secretion of TNF-α. Gadolinium chloride exposure was accompanied by changes in protease secretion from Kupffer cells and stellate cells, remodeling of the extracellular matrix, and repopulation of liver macrophages. Cholestasis and hyperbilirubinemia in ANIT-treated rats had similar characteristic (Ferreira et al., 2003) as in mice. In general, this process was more significant than the signs observed in patients with cholestasis due to medical treatment by different drugs (phenothiazine derivatives, methyltestosterone, estrogens, oral contraceptives, *etc.*). So, in experiment in mice and rats pretreatment with gadolinium chloride increased the severity of cholestasis and aggravated liver damage. Gadolinium accumulation in the liver (with peak after 24 h) was accompanied by a decrease in activity of proteases (cathepsin D and cathepsin B) and concentration of matrix metalloprotease-2 (Table 3) possibly, as a result of decreased liver macrophage number. Our observations confirm the hypothesis that normal function of Kupffer cells and extracellular matrix plays an important role in cholestasis. Administration of gadolinium chloride also serves as a convenient model to study the side effects, toxicity, and safety of lanthanides as nanoparticles.

The model of selective liver macrophage depression was characterized by decreased activity of serum chitotriosidase, whereas macrophage stimulation (by zymosan or chito-carboxymethyl β-1,3-glucans), on the contrary, increased chitotriosidase activity (Korolenko et al., 2008). The uptake of gadolinium by liver cells during preliminary (before gadolinium chloride) administration of β-1,3-glucans was also increased. It was suggested that the model of selective liver macrophage depression is useful for study the protective effects of different biological response modifiers such as polysaccharides (β-1,3-glucans) *in vivo.*

3.2 Liver injury and cholestasis

Bile duct obstruction, cholestasis development is associated with hepatic accumulation of leukocytes and liver injury (Gehring et al., 2006). According to our data obtained, the development of acute CCl_4-hepatitis was accompanied by hepatocyte cytolysis and increase in serum ALT activity (72 h after hepatotoxin administration to mice 9.50 ± 0.42, n=10 *vs* control 3.50 ± 0.29 U/L, n=10, $p < 0.01$), however cholestasis was not found in this model (no changes of alkaline phosphatase and GGTP activity in serum of mice comparatively to intact animals). During combined treatment by Triton WR 1339 and CCl_4 the cholestasis was more significant as compare to the group of mice received only Triton WR 1339. The aggravation of liver injury induced by Triton WR 1339, possibly, was related to increased damage of lysosomes by detergent and cholestasis development. It was shown in combined administration of Triton WR 1339+ CCl_4, that activity of β-galactosidase (116.8 ± 0.49 μmol MUF/L per min) and chitotriosidase (8.4 ± 0.55 μmol MUF/L per min) in bile was higher compared to intact mice (Table 2). The role of lysosomal enzymes in bile secretion in mice is still not clear. Previous studies showed that in intact mice "synchronous" exocytosis of lysosomal glucosidases (β-galactosidase, β-glucuronidase and N-acetyl-β-D-glucosaminidase) into bile occurred in intact rats (Korolenko et al., 2008). The function of lysosomal enzymes in the bile remains unclear. Glucosidases are probably involved into degradation of glucuronides. Dramatic increased in β-galactosidase activity and some changes in β-hexosaminidase and chitotriosidase in bile of mice with the both models of experimental cholestasis (induced by ANIT and Triton WR 1339) probably reflected the increased exocytosis of enzymes into bile. Transport disorders and concentration of lysosomal enzymes in bile can potentiate the effect of different compounds (lipids and fatty acids) excreted into bile independently of lysosomal enzymes. Hepatocytes and bile duct cells probably are connected with bile secretion in mice, but in general cellular source of lysosomal enzymes in bile and serum is not clear. The main part of plasma proteins in mammals (mice and rats) are synthesized in liver cells. In humans, serum chitotriosidase was shown to originate partially from macrophages and PMN, however in mice, on the contrary, chitotriosidase localized mainly in cells of the gastrointestinal mucosa (Korolenko et al., 2007; Aerts et al., 2008) and cellular source of this enzyme in serum and bile is still not clear.

3.3 Chitotriosidase activity in liver pathology

The special attention was devoted to chitotriosidase and intrahepatic cholestasis. Chitotriosidase is a new enzyme which was found in human macrophages (Aerts et al., 2008). There is limited information on the biological role of chitotriosidase in laboratoty animals (mice, rats, rabbits); as in humans, the main function of this enzyme is related to innate immunity. It was shown that serum chitotriosidase activity in patients with type I Gaucher disease increased up to 100-1000 times and now serves as a diagnostic surrogate marker of this disorder. In humans, enzyme activity markedly varies (9-195 nmol MUF/mL h) in healthy persons and increases with age (Aerts et al., 2008). Chitotriosidase activity is very low in 6.2% young individuals and high in 3.1% individuals. Enzyme activity moderately increases (by 2-3 times) in patients with inborn lysosomal storage diseases (Krabbe disease, GMI gangliosidose, and Niemann-Pick, type A and B disease). As was noted before, human chitotriosidase is mainly synthesized in macrophages; stimulated macrophages produce considerable amounts of chitotriosidase mRNA (Aerts et al., 2008). In neutrophil precursors chitotriosidase is synthesized and accumulated in specific granules. Chitin, a component of cell walls and membranes in various microorganisms, is the natural substrate for chitotriosidase; enzyme cleaves also the synthetic substrate 4-methylumbelliferyl-(MUF)-β-D-N,N',N''.-triacetylchitotrioside. Chitinases of plants protect them from various pathogenic fungi, this function is similar to mammalian chitotriosidase. Probably, mammalian chitotriosidase also has some protective properties. Functions of chitotriosidase need further studies. The role of this enzyme is connected with innate immunity and removing of foreign bacteria and fungi, whose membranes include chitin; this function of chitotriosidase is of particular interest. In mammals, the biological function of *serum* chitotriosidase, as well as its cell origin in experimental lysosomal storage syndrome, is poor understood (possibly, enzyme is originated from the stimulated macrophages). Earlier we have shown the increase of chitotriosidase activity in serum of experimental animals (mice and rats) in macrophage stimulation (by zymosan, carboxymethyl β-glucan), which were taken up by Kupffer cells and stimulate liver macrophages and also lung and spleen macrophage pools. Triton WR-1339 administration in mice was shown to increase the number of liver macrophages and reproduce lysosomal storage syndrome, elevating serum chitotriosidase activity 5-7 days after the single drug administration. Thus, macrophage stimulation by β-glucans, Triton WR 1339 moderately (1.5-2-times) increased serum chitotriosidase activity in experimental animals (mice and rats). However, in these experimental models stimulation of macrophages in rats and mice did not dramatically increase chitotriosidase activity as in type I Gaucher disease in human serum (i.e. more than by 100-1000-times).

β-Hexosaminidase is one of glucosidase, which had been studied earlier in serum of humans and mice. However, there is limited number of works devoted to secretion of this enzyme into bile (possibly, by exocytosis). The most of investigations were devoted to study this enzyme in humans. Human plasma contains a high-molecular weight enzyme precursor (63kDa) of β-hexosaminidase A and B. The presence of 38 kDa mature enzymes in liver lysosomes of mammals is related to processing inside of these particles. The bile of mice probably contains mature β-hexosaminidase, which is secreted by exocytosis after enzyme processing in lysosomes.

The development of cholestasis in humans and experimental animals may be also associated with metabolic disorders of lipids and lipoproteins and accompanies liver injury of different etiology. Releasing of lysosomal enzymes can increase the severity of hepatocyte damage under the influence of toxic components from the bile (fatty acids salts), which can exert modulatory effect on apoptosis of liver cells. Administration of ANIT is rapidly (8-24 h after) followed by reversible damage of the epithelium of bile ducts and serves as a widely used model of intrahepatic cholestasis in rats and mice. Macrophage depression by gadolinium chloride aggravated the cholestasis development in mice induced by ANIT.

Preliminary administration of Triton WR 1339 in mice and rats, aggravated the development of acute toxic hepatitis induced by CC_4. The development of CCl_4-induced hepatitis (after 72 h) was accompanied by hepatocyte cytolysis and increase in plasma ALT activity (9.50±0.42 U/L per h, n=10; *vs.* 3.50±0.29 U/L per h in the control, n=10; p<0.01). Cholestasis in acute toxic hepatitis was not found under isolated CCl_4 administration in mice. However, aggravation of cholestasis and especially, liver injury was observed after preliminary administration of Triton WR 1339 to mice with acute toxic hepatitis. The aggravation of cholestasis after combined treatment by Triton WR 1339 and CCl_4 was probably associated with effect of Triton WR 1339 on liver lysosomes. Activities of β-galactosidase (116.80± 0.49 μmol MUF/L per min, n=5) and chitotriosidase (8.40±0.55 μmol MUF/L per min in bile samples from treated animals were significantly higher compared to intact mice and animals with isolated administration of Triton WR 1339.

4. Conclusion

Intrahepatic cholestasis was shown to develop during treatment by different medical drugs (antibiotics, phenothiazine derivaties, anti-inflammatory drugs), some of them possessed by lysosomotropic action (these drugs are taken up and selectively concentrated *in vivo* inside of lysosomes). The lysosomotropic action of drugs was shown in medical clinics using some antibiotics, iron compounds. In experiment we compared the cholestasis development in mice with help of known ANIT model and lysosomotropic agent Triton WR 1339 administration. We compared these models to reveal the common features of intrahepatic cholestasis, during study of bile and serum enzymes in animals with intrahepatic cholestasis. Intrahepatic cholestasis development was confirmed by elevation of serum alkaline phosphatase and γ-glutamyl transferase activity in the both cases. According to morphological (electron microscopic) study of liver cells enlargement of bile canaliculi and bile ducts was noted as well as other morphological signs of intrahepatic cholestasis. Both models of intrahepatic cholestasis can be used for reproduction in mice (and rats). It was concluded that drug-induced intrahepatic cholestasis is manifested in increased secretion of lysosomal enzymes into the bile. Bile components can aggravate liver cells damage by affecting the process of hepatocyte apoptosis and necrosis. Selective depression of Kupffer cells, enriched by lysososomes, reproduced *in vivo* (with help of gadolinium chloride) was followed by the aggravation of cholestasis and liver damage. Our results confirm the hypothesis that normal function of liver macrophages and their lysosomes play the important role in cholestasis development. These data can be useful in further investigation of the role of lysosomes of hepatocytes and liver macrophages in bile secretion and, possibly, in prevention of cholestasis development in medical clinics used some drugs with lysosomotropic action (phenothiazines, some antibiotics, polymers, iron compound, chloroquine etc.).

5. Acknowledgement

Authors are grateful to senior researcher of the Institute of Cytology and Genetic Siberian Branch of Russian Academy of Sciences (Novosibirsk) Dr. Kaledin V.I. for kind help in providing experiments with ANIT; Dr. Zhanaeva S.Y. for assay of cysteine protease activity in liver of mice with gadolinium chloride administration, Dr. Klishevich M.S. , Dr. Goncharova I.A., Dr. Cherkanova M.S. for help.

6. References

Abe, C., Ikeda, S., Uchida, T., Yamashita, K., & Ichikawa, T. (2007). Triton WR 1339, an inhibitor of lipoprotein lipase, decreases vitamin E concentration in some tissues of rats by inhibiting its transport to liver./*J. Nutr.*/, Vol. 137, No. 2, (Feb 2007), pp. 345-350, ISSN 0022-3166; Online ISSN 1541-6100.

Aerts, J.M., van Breemen, M.J., Bussink, A.P., Ghauharali, K., Sprenger, R., Boot, R.G., Groener, J.E., Hollak, C.E., Maas, M., Smit, S., Hoefsoot, H.C., Smilde, A.K., Vissers, J.P. de Jong, S., Speijer D., & de Koster, C.G. (2008). Biomarkers for lysosomal storage disorders: identification and application as exemplified by chitotriosidase in Gaucher disease. /*Acta Paediatr. Suppl.*/,Vol. 97, No.457 (Apr 2008), pp. 7-14. ISSN 0803-5326 (Print) ; 0803-5326 (Linking).

Chandra, P., & Brouwer K.L.R. (2004). The complexities of hepatic drug transport: current knowledge and emerging concepts. 2004. /*Pharmaceutical Research*/, Vol. 21, No. 5, (May 2004), pp.719-735, ISSN 0724-8741 (print version) ISSN 1573-904X (electronic version)

Chang, M.-L., Yeh, C.-T., Chang, P.-Y., & Chen, J.-C. (2005). Comparison of murine cirrhosis models induced by hepatotoxin administration and common bile duct ligation. /*World J. Gastroenterol.*/, 2005, Vol. 11, No. 27, (Jul 2005), pp. 4167-4172, ISSN 1007-9327

de Duve, C., de Barsy, T., Poole., B, Trouet, A., Tulkens, P., & Van /Hoof, F. Comments. Lysosomotropic agents. (1974). /*Biochem. Pharmacol.*/,Vol. 23, No. 18, (Sept. 1974), pp.2495-2531, ISSN 0006-2952.

Dergunova, M.A., Alexeenko, T.V., Zhanaeva, S.Y., Filjushina, E.E., Buzueva I.I., Kolesnikova, O.P., Kogan, G., & Korolenko. T.A. Characterization of the novel chemically modified fungal polysaccharides as the macrophage stimulators. (2009). /*Int. Immunopharmacol.* /, Vol. 9, No. 6, (Jun 2009), pp.729-733. ISSN 1567-5769.

Ding H., Peng R., Reed E., Li Q.Q. Effects of Kupffer cell inhibition on liver function and hepatocellular activity in mice. (2003). *Int. J./ Mol. Med.*/, Vol. 12, No. 4 (Oct. 2003), pp. 549-557, ISSN 1791-244X.

Dold, S., Laschke, M.W., Lavasani, S., Menger, M.D., Jeppsson, B., & Thorlacius, H. (2009). Simvastatin protects against cholestasis-induced liver injury. /*Br. J. Pharmacol.*/, Vol. 156, No.3, (Feb 2009), pp. 466-474, ISSN 0007-1188

Ferreira, F.M., Oliveira, P.J., Rolo, A.P., Santos, M.S., Moreno, A.J., da Cunha, M.F., Seica, R. & Palmeira, C.M. (2003). Cholestasis induced by chronic treatment with alpha-naphtyl-isothiocyanate (ANIT) affects rat renal mitochondrial bioenergetics. /*Arch. Toxicol.*/, Vol. 77, No. 4, (Apr 2003), pp.194-200. ISSN: 0340-5761. ISSN: 1432-0738 (electronic version).

Gehring, S., Dickson, E.M, San Martin, M.E., van Rooijen, N., Papa, E.F., Harty, M.W, Tracy, TF.Jr & Gregory, S.H.(2006). Kupffer cells abrogate cholestatic liver injury in mice. /*Gastroenterology*/, Vol. 130, No. 3, (March 2006), pp. 810-822. ISSN: 0016-5085.

Hoffmann, A.F. (2002). Cholestatic liver disease: pathophysiology and therapeutic options. /*Liver*/, Vol. 22, Suppl. 2, (2002). pp.14-19, ISSN: 0106-9543

Hsien, C.-S., Huang, C.-C., Huang L.-T., Chung, J.-C., & Chou M.-H. 2006. Reversible cholestasis and cholangitis induced by biliary drainage and infusion in the rat. /*Eur. Surg. Res.* /, Vol. 38, No. 1, (Feb 2006), pp. 11-17, ISSN (printed): 0014-312X. ISSN (electronic) 1421-9921

Jansen, P..L., & Sturm, E. (2003). Genetic cholestasis causes and consequences for hepatobiliary transport. /*Liver Int.* /, Vol. 23, No. 5, (Oct 2003), pp.315-322, ISSN 1478-3223

Kodali, P., Wu, P., Lahiji, P.A., Brown, E.J., & Maher, J.J. (2006). ANIT toxicity toward mouse hepatocytes *in vivo* is mediated primary by neutrophyls via CD18. /*Am. J. Physiol. Gastrointest Liver Physiol.*/, Vol..291, No. 2, (Aug 2006), pp. G355-G363, ISSN: 0193-1857

Korolenko, T.A., Goncharova, I.A., Anterejkina, L.I., Levina, O.A. & Korolenko, C.P. (2007). Influence of opiate addiction on liver cell damage of patients with viral hepatitis C. /*Alaska Med.* /, Vol.49, No. 2 Suppl., (2007), pp. 75-78, ISSN #0002-4538

Korolenko, T.A., Savchenko, N.G., Yuz'ko, Ju.V., Alexeenko, T.V., & Sorochinskaya, N.V. (2008). Activity of lysosomal enzymes in the bile and serum of mice with intrahepatic cholestasis. /*Bull. Exper. Biol. Med.*/, Vol.145, No. 5, (May 2008), pp. 560-563. ISSN (electronic) 1573-8221

Korolenko, T.A., Cherkanova, M.S., Tuzikov, F.V., Johnston, T.P., Tuzikova, N.A., Loginova, V.M., & Kaledin, V.I. (2011). Influence of atorvastatin on fractional and subfractional composition of serum lipoproteins and MMP activity in mice with Triton WR 1339-induced lipemia. /*J. Pharm. Pharmacol.*/, Vol. 63, No 6 (June 2011), pp.833-839, ISSN: 0022-3573

Krell, H., Metz, J., Jaeschke. H., Hoke, H., & Pfaff, E. Drug-induced intrahepatic cholestasis: characterization of different pathomechanisms. (1987). /*Arch. Toxicol.*/, Vol. 60, No. 1-3, pp.124-130. ISSN (printed): 0340-5761. ISSN (electronic): 1432-0738.

Luyendyk, J.P., Mackman, N. & Sullivan, B.P. (2011). Role of fibrinogen and protease-activated receptors in acute xenobiotic-induced cholestatic liver injury. /*Toxicol. Sci.*/, Vol. 119, No. 1, (Jan. 2011), pp. 233-243. ISSN 1015-1621.

Meier, P.J., & Stieger, B. (2000). Molecular mechanisms of bile formation. /*News Physiol. Sci.*/, Vol.15, No. 2, (Apr. 2000), pp. 89-93, ISSN (printed): 0886-1714

Moritoki, Y., Ueno, Y., Kanno, N., Yamagiwa, Y., Fukushima, K., Gershwin, M.E. & Shimosegawa, T. (2006). Lack of evidence that bone marrow cells contribute to cholangiocyte repopulation during experimental cholestatic ductal hyperplasia. /Liver International/, Vol. 26, No. 4, (May 2006), pp. 457-466, ISSN: 1478-3223

Paumgartner, G. (2006). Medical treatment of cholestatic liver diseases: from pathobiology to pharmacological targets. /*World J. Gastroenterol.*/, Vol. 12, No. 28, (Jul 2008), pp.4445-4451, ISSN 1007-9327

Rodriguez-Garay, E.A. (2003). Cholestasis: human disease and experimental animal models. /*Ann. Hepatol.*/, Vol. 2, No 4, (Oct-Dec 2003), pp.150-158, ISSN: 1665-2681

Sherlock, S. & Dooley, J. (1997). Cholestasis. In: Diseases of the liver and biliary system, 10th eds. Blackwell Science Inc., Malde, MA, pp. 217-237.

Schneider, P., Korolenko, T.A., & Busch, U. A review of drug-induced lysosomal disorders of the liver in man and laboratory animals. /*Microsc. Res. Tech.* /, Vol. 36, No. 4, (Feb 1997), pp. 253-275, ISSN (printed): 1059-910X. ISSN (electronic): 1097-0029

Trout, J.J. & Viles, J.M. Cellular changes associated with triton WR-1339 accumulation in rat liver hepatocytes. II. Lysosomal triton WR-1339 accumulation. (1979). /*Exp. Mol. Pathol.*/, Vol.31, No.1 (Aug. 1979), pp.81-90, ISSN 0014-4800.

5

Phytosterols and Lack of Occurrence of Cholestasis in Rats Nourished Parenterally or Orally

M.L. Forchielli et al.*,**
Pediatrics, S'Orsola-Malpighi, Bologna Medical School, Italy

1. Introduction

Intravenous lipid emulsions (ILEs) have been marketed to infuse fat within total parenteral nutrition (TPN) in order to prevent essential fatty acid deficiency. Only recently, ILEs have been recognized to have therapeutic effects in gastrointestinal, cardiovascular, pulmonary, oncologic, autoimmune, and critical care diseases. At the same time, toxic substances such as phytosterols have been found in ILEs. Phytosterols have been related to a TPN-associated complication defined parenteral nutrition-associated cholestasis (PNAC) (1-5).

In a previous study (6), we found phytosterols to be considerably present in all the lipid emulsions analyzed so as to exceed the amount physiologically absorbed by the gut. In this study, we want to determine the plasma amount of phytosterols deriving from different oil sources in rats receiving parenteral nutrition, and compare it with those in rats on standard oral diet. Subsequently, we want to verify whether phytosterols have an impact on the occurrence of cholestasis. Finally, we intend to verify whether the addition of glutamine changes the outcomes.

Phytosterols, cholesterol, intravenous lipid emulsions, cholestasis, gas chromatography

ILEs: intravenous lipid emulsions
PNAC: parenteral nutrition-associated cholestasis
IL: parenteral nutrition with soy bean oil
TPN : total parenteral nutrition
ILG: parenteral nutrition with soy bean oil plus glutamine
CTR: standard control
ALT : alanine aminotransferase
ALKP : alkaline phosphatase

* G. Bersani[2], S. Tala'[3], G. Grossi[3], A. Munarini[3], L. Martini[4], C. Puggioli[2], R. Giardino[4] and A. Pession [1]
[1]*Paediatrics, S.Orsola-Malpighi Medical School*
[2]*Pharmacy Service*
[3]*Chemical Laboratory, S.Orsola-Malpighi*
[4]*Experimental Surgery, Rizzoli Research Institute, Bologna Medical School, Italy*
** Corresponding author

GC : gas chromatography
SD: standard deviation

2. Materials and methods

2.1 Animal experiments

Animal and plant sterols were quantified in the plasma of fifteen 7-week-old genetically inbred male Wistar rats (Charles River, Calco, Como, Italy), divided in three groups: one group was infused with TPN containing Intralipid® (Fresenius Kabi AG, Germany) as lipid emulsion (IL), a second group received the same regimen with the addition of glutamine (15% of total amino acid composition) (ILG), and the third group was fed chow and served as standard control (CTR). PN was daily injected intraperitoneally for 5 days. Diets were isocalorical and their gross energy density was 10 kcal/die, divided into protein 20, lipid 40 and carbohydrate 40 in case of TPN and 5% fats (from soy), 20% proteins, and the remaining carbohydrates from chow. The animals, housed in individual room with controlled temperature and light conditions, had open access to food (Mucedola 2518; Settimo Milanese, Milan, Italy). They were allowed to acclimatize to these conditions for a week, then they were randomly divided into the three groups. Animal care, housing and killing met the guidelines of the Italian Health Ministry, which approved the study. Rats were weighted at the beginning of the study and before being killed. In the fifth day the animals were killed and their blood and liver samples were taken. Some blood samples were sent to the laboratory to determine liver function tests, lipid profile, and bile acids by enzymatic method, while others were collected in Eppendorf with EDTA and stored at - 80°C until analysis. Some liver samples (4–6 µm) were fixed in 10% neutral buffered formalin for 48 h, embedded in paraffin, and stained with hematoxylin and eosin prior to microscopic examination.

2.2 Reagents, solvents, and standards

Chloroform (analytical reagent grade), *n*-hexane (analytical reagent grade), methanol (Lichrosolv), diethyl ether, anhydrous sodium sulphate, potassium chloride, and potassium hydroxide were supplied by Merck (Darmstadt, Germany). Acetone (AnalaR®) was purchased from BDH (VWR International Ltd., Leicestershire, UK). Bidistilled water and silylating agents (pyridine, hexamethyldisilazane and trimethylchlorosilane) were supplied by Carlo Erba (Milano, Italy). (24*R*)-ethylcholest-5-en-3β-ol (β-sitosterol) purity: 60% β-sitosterol and 30% (24*R*)-methylcholest-5-en-3β-ol (campesterol) was purchased from Research Plus (Bayonne, NJ, USA). (24*S*)-Ethylcholest-5,22-dien-3β-ol (stigmasterol) (purity: 93%), cholest-5-en-3β-ol (cholesterol) (purity: 99%), and 5α-cholestane (purity: 97%) were purchased from Sigma (St. Louis, MO, USA). The purity of the standards was controlled by gas chromatography (GC).

2.3 Quantification of sterols

Lipid extraction and sterol determination were performed in plasma by a technique which processes were shown in tables 1.

Plasma levels were quantified ***by Gas chromatography-mass spectrometry*** technique according to ***Cold trapping technique,*** *"solvent vent injection"* mode.
Sample pretreatment ***Sample dilution:*** rat plasma sample 50 µl in sterile saline 50 µl (1:1 dilution). ***Internal standard solution:*** 5α-cholestane in ethanol 1.26 ± 0.06 mg/ml. ***Sterol standard solution:*** mixed of cholesterol/cholestanol/campesterol/stigmasterol/sitosterol in ethanol 2958 ± 0.6/384 ± 0.2/0.77 ± 231 ± 0.2/60 ± 0.2/302 ± 0.2 µg/300 µl respectively. ***Saponification*** and ***extraction procedure:*** sample 100 µl + "work" internal standard 1 ml (internal standard in diethylether/tetrametilammonium hydroxide/isopropanol (1:13:36 v/v/v) - *Incubation* at 80°C for 15 min - *Extraction* by tetrachloroethylene/methylbuthyrate 500 µl (1:3 v/v) and sterile water 2 ml. Organic phase exsiccation under nitrogen flow and derivatization with Tri-Sil® silyling mixture at 60°C for an hour.
Gas chromatography conditions ***Injection volume:*** extracted solution 2 µl. ***Gas chromatograph:*** GC HP 5890 Agilent with autosampler. ***Gas carrier:*** highly purified helium. ***Flow rate:*** 0.5 ml/min. ***Column conditions:*** capillary column HP-5MS, 5% PH SM Siloxane Crosslinked, heated from 100° C to 280° C for 21 min. ***Detector: mass spectroscope*** MS 5973 Agilent. ***Oven temperature:*** 60°C ***Software:*** HP 5973N, rev D002 for data registration, integration and treatment. ***Assay validation:*** specificity, detection and quantitation limit, linearity, precision and accuracy. Every sample was triple-tested.

Table 1. Determination of sterols

2.4 Data analysis

Results were summarized according to distribution in mean and standard deviation (SD) or median and range. Comparisons of means among experiments groups were carried out using a 1-tailed analysis of variance test with multiple-comparison tests using the Bonferroni option to compare plasma sterol contents among groups. Comparisons of medians were performed using the Kruskal Wallis and Wilcoxon test for non parametric data. Statistical tests were performed using the STATA Software 11 (Santa Monica, California). Then, the results were associated with the liver specimens, which were read by two different pathologists, both blinded to the type of nourishment received by the rats and unaware of each other's opinion. Statistical differences were considered significant at a p-value of <0.05.

3. Results

All animals behaved normally during the study. They all gained weights and there was non significant differences among groups during the study. Summary of descriptive data is summarized in table 2. Serum liver function tests were determined as marker of liver alteration. Total and direct bilirubin, cholesterol, and biliary acid were averagely normal and they not differed among groups. Alanine aminotransferase (ALT) and alkaline phosphatase (ALKP) reached a statistically difference. Noteworthy, both had a higher level in the control group than the others' receiving TPN. Also glucose (not reached a significant difference), along with bile acids were increased in the control group as compared to the other two. Trygliceriedes (p value= 0.05 borderline) were highly represented in the ILG group. Upon collection, livers were noted to be dark red in all groups and their weights were similar.

	IL	ILG	Control	p-value
Weight delta gr, (median/range)	20 (5-25)	15 (5-20)	20 (5-25)	NS
ALT U/L (median/range)	39 (25-69)	31 (13-41)	56 (45-201)	0.018
ALKP U/L (median/range)	338 (69-510)[A]	388 (276-426)[B]	578 (505-657)	0.016
Glucose mg/dl (median/range)	264 (233-312)	352 (278-407)	444 (303-464)	NS
Total bili mg/dl (median/range)	0.08 (0.07-2.55)	0.03 (0.03-0.03)	0.12 (0.06-0.17)	NS
Direct bili mg/dl (median/range)	0.02 (0.02-0-03)	0.045 (0.02-0-05)	0.04 (0.03-0.04)	NS
Bile acids micromol/dl (median/range)	12.3 (9.2-12.6)	5.7 (5.2-6.5)	13.6 (5.2-56.8)	NS
Trygliceriedes mg/dl (median/range)	98.5 (79-2691)	303 (55-428)	65 (28-82)	0.05
Cholesterol mg/dl (median/range)	90 (29-140)	85 (67-136)	92 (66-103)	NS

ALKP: alkaline phosphatase
ALT: alanine aminotransferase

- [A]:p value= 0.027 compared to control group
- [B]: p value= 0.009 compared to control group

Table 2. Summary of the descriptive data

The lipids were quantified and classified by type of sterols (animal: cholesterol, and plant: β-sitosterol, campesterol, and stigmasterol). Table 3 summarizes the total amount of sterols given to rats on parenteral nutrition. Table 4 summarizes the amount of lipids extracted from plasma and figure 1 shows their plasma concentrations. Animal and plant sterols were differently infused in the animals, with the latter generally accounting for a greater share than the former. Conversely, the same animal and plant sterols were inversely represented with cholesterol content largely predominant in the plasma of rats. Among phytosterols, sitosterol had the highest plasma level in all the groups. Its highest concentrations were found in the ILG group, followed by the IL group. Controls had the lowest content, which, however, was not significant as differences among groups were not statistically significant. Plasma stigmasterol levels were significantly higher in both the IL and ILG groups. This time, differences were statistically significant ($p=0.000$). With respect to stigmasterol, a multiple pairwise comparison among groups confirmed a borderline statistically significant pairwise differences between IL and the control group (p:0.068). Plasma campesterol levels were similar across groups including the one receiving chow and differences were not significant.

Rat groups	Cholesterol (mg)	Campesterol (mg)	Stigmasterol (mg)	Sitosterol (mg)	Plant Sterol (mg)	Plant Sterol + Cholesterol (mg)
IL	3.0	0.68	0.72	2.5	3.9	6.8
ILG	2.72	0.60	0.64	2.9	3.5	6.2

Table 3. Overall amount of sterols parenterally injected into the rats

Rat group	Cholesterol mean (μg/ml)	Colestanol mean ±SD (μg/ml)	Campesterol mean ± SD (μg/ml)	Stigmasterol mean ± SD (μg/ml)	Sitosterol mean ± SD (μg/ml)	Total (μg/ml)
IL	>20.0	0.10 ± 0.1	0.9 ± 0.3	0.11 ± 0.01*	1.80 ± 0.3	22.91
ILG	>20.0	0.12 ± 0.04	0.7 ± 0.2	0.10 ± 0.1	1.50 ± 0.6	22.46
Chow	>20.0	0.20 ± 0.1	0.9 ± 0.2	0.014 ± 0.003	1.30 ± 0.5	22.41

*:p value= 0.068 when comparing IL with chow

Table 4. Quantification of plasma level of sterols in rats receiving parenteral, or oral nourishment

After regressing the amounts of provided sterols to the plasma levels identified, a strong positive association was found for the stigmasterol ($R^2=0.83$). Weaker associations were found for campesterol ($R^2=0.37$) and sitosterol ($R^2=0.34$).

None of the liver specimens showed abnormalities. Normal hepatic architecture and no evidence of PNAC or hepatic steatosis were found in all groups. Minor derangements were seen in scattered sections with signs of hepatic hypoxia around the central vein regions, which were likely due to the animal's sacrifice.

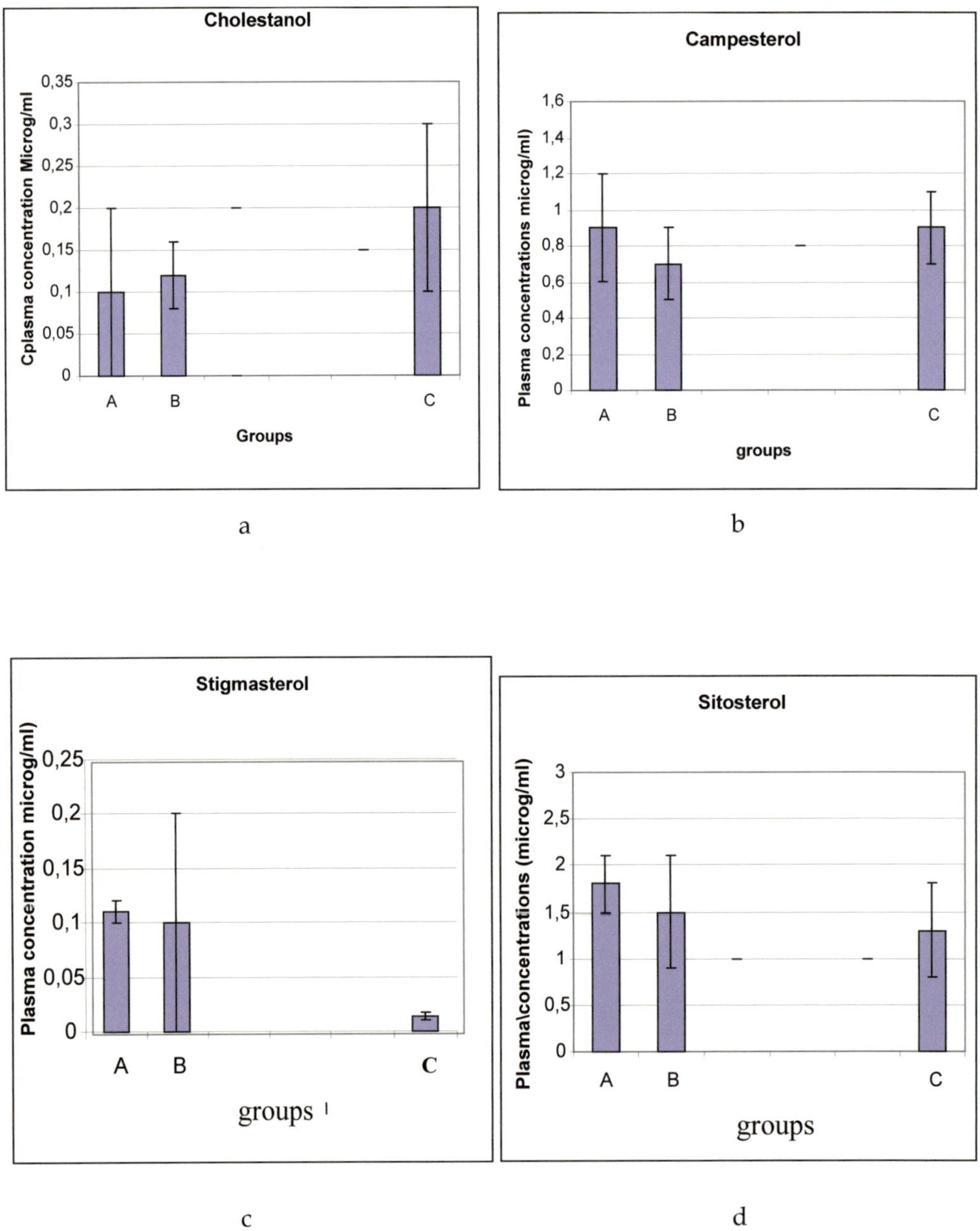

Fig. 1. Plasma concentrations of sterols

4. Discussion

Scattered reports in the literature have linked PNAC to the vegetable sterol components of ILEs (1-5). Information on the sterol contents of ILEs, however, is currently scant and one of our previous purpose was to identify animal and plant sterols contained in the most representative ILEs. To this end, we selected ILE formulations as being representative in terms of their main oil component (soy, olive oil, fish oil variably combined with medium- or long-chain fatty acids, and purified triglycerides) and we quantified their animal and vegetal sterol contents (6). The relative weight of each sterol, however, varied significantly across formulations, but cholesterol and beta-sitosterol were the most represented followed by campesterol and stigmasterol. Our second hypothesis was then to verify the distribution of these sterols into plasma of rats and check their effects on liver structure. Therefore, in this study, we divided inbred weaning rats in three groups (two groups receiving TPN with or without glutamine and the third receiving chow) and we determined how sterols were distributed in plasma. Rats' liver status was also checked to verify whether sterols have changed histology in the short term.

While animal and vegetal sterols were differently represented across ILEs, with the latter generally present in greater amounts than the former, the opposite occurred in the plasma of rats regardless of their original nourishment. Cholesterol content was largely predominant in all groups, followed by sitosterol. Sitosterol was higher in those receiving TPN, although its level did not significantly differ among groups and did not correlate with the amount supplied. Campesterol was similarly represented in all three groups, while stigmasterol which had the lowest levels, was significantly correlated with the amount supplemented, and was even more significantly represented in the IL and ILG groups (p value 0.000). While expected in the TPN groups, it was a surprise to have found plant sterols considerably present in the plasma of rats fed with chow, given that sterols are usually not absorbed by the gastrointestinal system. As in humans, plasma concentrations of plant sterols, all detectable at low concentrations, vary at the individual level due to genetic polymorphism, it is possible that similar processes occur in animals. β-sitosterol, which is not endogenously produced, is rapidly secreted as neutral sterol into bile more than cholesterol and other plant sterols (9). This more rapid fractional turnover of β-sitosterol may indirectly indicate that the rigorous exclusion of sterols other than cholesterol in vertebrates may be essential for the maintenance of normal cholesterol homeostasis. When mutations affect the heterodimers transporter complex, sitosterolemia and hypercholesterolemia occur and atherosclerosis may develop. This process was highlighted in homologous animal proteins (10,11).

The association between phytosterols and PNAC has not been confirmed in this study carried out over a short term infusion of a high lipid load (40% vs 7 % of fat present in chow). These results are in contrast with those from other studies. La Scala et al, for instance, showed a direct correlation between the addition of lipids and the development of PNAC, which occurred in rats after 3 days of TPN infusion (5). On the contrary, Romestaing et al. proved that a long term highly saturated fat diet did not induce steatohepatitis in rats, but rather increased peripheral fat storage and thermogenesis (12). Interestingly, laboratory data obtained in our study, showed better parameters in the groups receiving ILEs' as compared to those in controls. Even though our original idea was to find an association between TPN and liver dysfunction, this finding would go to an opposite direction and be a sign of ILEs' protection. The ILG group has the lowest GPT level as if the addition of glutamine had preserved hepatic functions. As previously reported in the literature, glutamine preserves liver glutathione after acute injuries and is able to cleanse the liver of the waste products (13). That is why we could have not found any histological alterations in the liver. The mechanisms through which phytosterols allegedly activate or, more precisely, influence or contribute to a cholestatic process in the liver are obscure. Perhaps the multifactorial origin of PNAC does not allow to separately assess the effects of each risk factor. Bypassing the gastrointestinal system, a high load of vegetal sterols with ILEs easily overload the blood stream and the liver. On top of the infused cholesterol, it is possible that both sterols act sinergically or competitively with the liver transporter system, which may displace either vegetal or animal sterol excretions and lead to bile duct plugging and initial inflammation. With continuous infusion of these sterols, infections, lack of oral intake, multiple drugs use, and surgery, the process might worsen. The finding that a patient developed a cirrhosis secondary to an autoimmune hepatitis and the combined occurrence of sitosterolemia due to a compound heterozygote ABCG8 gene mutation, may reflect a two-hit step and explain the need for liver transplantation, which completely reversed the phytosterol storage (14).

Stigmasterol was the only plant sterol which differentiated the three animal groups. A recent study investigating the role of different phytosterols (sitosterol, campesterol, and stigmasterol) in the induction of liver damage has shown that stigmasterol is a potent antagonist of the nuclear farnesoid X receptor FXR and the ligand-activated pregnane X receptor (a member also of the NR superfamily involved in the bile acid metabolism and inflammation), while sitosterol and campesterol had minimal or insignificant inhibitory effects in a human-derived liver cell line HepG2 (15). In addition to the agonist action of the liver X receptors (LXRs) (highly expressed in the liver, adipose tissue, intestine, kidney, and macrophages with involvement in sterol transport, fatty acid metabolism, glucose regulation, immunity , and cellular response), stigmasterol also interferes with the processing of sterol response element binding protein-2 (SREBP-2), which is a central regulatory factor in cholesterol metabolism. The nuclear receptor (NR) superfamily has been targeted as the main regulator in the adaptive response to cholestasis. In particular, the FXR NR1H4 seems to be the key regulator of intrahepatic bile acid levels. To maintain safe levels, it reprograms hepatic transcriptional factors reducing sinusoidal bile acid import, suppressing bile acid synthesis, and increasing intrahepatic bile acid efflux across canalicular and sinusoidal membranes. When FXR NR1H4 is lacking, hepatocytes are more susceptible to bile acid-induced injuries in rats. These rats, conversely, do not develop cholestasis if FXR NR1H4 is added back (16). Other studies have shown that phytosterols inhibit cholesterol 7-α-hydroxylase, which is the rate-limiting step for the conversion of cholesterol into bile acids (17). The mechanism by which stigmasterol disrupts cholesterol homeostasis activating LXR and suppressing the SREBP pathway was experimentally probed in a study in vitro where the authors also identified other sterols such as desmosterol, a cholesterol precursor (18). Apparently a double bond in the side chain of the sterol structure is responsible for the activation of LXR. Whether ILEs with high content of stigmasterol are crucial in the development of PNAC is yet to be proven. However, we believe that the solution's key lays in the interaction between phytosterols and phospholipids as proven in a model study in which the effect of the sterols on the molecular organization of the phospholipid monolayers was analyzed based on the compression modulus values (19). It was found that the incorporation of the phytosterols into the phospholipid monolayers increased their condensation, without affecting the stoichiometry of the most stable phospholipids complexes. However, their stability was greatly affected. Cholesterol/phospholipids mixtures had the strongest interactions, while systems containing stigmasterol had the weakest.

The use of the intraperitoneal route to infuse TPN could be another explanation for the lack of hepatic derangements in this study. The intraperitoneal route is a well established procedure to infuse fluids and drugs in rodents (20). We decided to use the intraperitoneal route to avoid inserction of an central venous line, which would have exposed animals to two of the risk factors involved in the development of hepatic injuries: anesthesia and development of central venous line infections. Both factors would have greatly contributed to confuse the final outcome, due to the brief time of observation we planned. The intraperitoneal route was effective as the animals did not develop infections and were free to move without restrains.

One final thought goes to the selection of rats used in this study. To reduce the variability from selection bias, we decided to use inbred rats. In this way, differences could be totally attributed to the various feeding types as opposed to the inherited patterns of animals.

In conclusion phytosterols, which predominate in the infused ILEs compared to cholesterol, seem to be present in the plasma in quantities lower than cholesterol. No liver histological alterations occurred after a short-term high-fat parenteral infusions. These determinations will require further confirmation in long-term TPN supplementation and need to be analyzed taking into consideration the distribution of animal and plant sterols in the liver along with production of oxysterols.

5. References

[1] Bindl, L., D. Lütjohann, S. Buderus, M.J. Lentze, K.V. Bergmann. (2000). High plasma levels of phytosterols in patients on parenteral nutrition: a marker of liver dysfunction. J Pediatr Gastr Nutr. 31:313-6.

[2] Llop, J.M., N. Virgili, J.M. Moreno-Villares, P. García-Peris, T. Serrano, M. Forga, J. Solanich, A.M. Pita. (2008). Phytosterolemia in parenteral nutrition patients: Implications for liver disease development. Nutrition. 24:1145-52.

[3] Clayton, P.T., A. Bowron, K.A. Mills, A Massoud, M Casteels, PJ Milla. (1993). Phytosterolemia in children with parenteral nutrition-associated cholestatic liver disease. Gastroenterology. 105:1806-13.

[4] Iyer, K.R., P. Clayton. (19980. New insight into mechanisms of parenteral nutrition-associated cholestasis: role of plant sterols. J Pediatr Surg. 33:1-6.

[5] Lascala, G.C., C. Le Coultre, B.G. Roche, et al. (1993). The addition of lipids increases the TPN-associated cholestasis in the rat. Eur J Pediatr Surg. 3:224-7.

[6] Forchielli, M.L., G. Bersani, S. Tala', G. Grossi, C. Puggioli, M. Masi. (2010). The spectrum of plant and animal sterols in different oil-derived intravenous emulsions. Lipids. 45:63-71.

[7] Ishikawa, T.T., J. MacGee, J.A. Morrison, C.J. Glueck. (1974). Quantitative analysis of cholesterol in 5 to 20 µl of plasma. J Lipid Research. 15:286-91.

[8] Beaty, T.H., P.O. Kwiterovich Jr, M.J. Khoury, S. White, P.S. Bachorik, H.H. Smith, B. Teng, A. Sniderman. (1986). Genetic analysis of plasma sitosterol, apoprotein B, and

lipoproteins in a large Amish pedigree with sitosterolemia. Am J Hum Genet. 38:492-504.
[9] Salen G, Ahrens EH, Grundy SM (1970) Metabolism of β-sitosterol in men. J Clin Invest 49:952-67.
[10] Graf GA, Yu L, Li WP, et al. (2003) ABCG5 and ABCG8 are obligate heterodimers for protein trafficking and biliary cholesterol excretion. J Biol Chem 278:48275-82.
[11] Wang J, Zhang D, Lei Y, et al. (2008) Purification and reconstitution of sterol transfer by native mouse ABCG5 and ABCG8. Biochemistry 47:5194-204.
[12] Romestaing C, Piquet MA, Bedu E, Rouleau V, Dautresme M, Hourmand-Ollivier I, Filippi C, Duchamp C, Sibille B. (2007) Long term highly saturated fat diet does not induce NASH in Wistar rats. Nutrition & Metabolism;4:1-14 doi 10.1186/1743-7075-4-4.
[13] Yu JC, Jiang ZM, Li DM. Glutamine: a precursor of glutathione and its effects on liver. Worl J Gastr 1999;5:143-6.
[14] Miettinen TA, Klett EL, Gylling H, Isoniemi H, Patel SB (2006) Liver transplantation in a patient with sitosterolemia and cirrhosis. Gastroenterology 130:542-7.
[15] Carter BA, Taylor OA, Prendergast DR, et al. (2007) Stigmasterol, a so lipid-derived phytosterol, is an antagonist of the bile acid nuclear receptor FXR. Pediatr Res 62:301-6.
[16] Liu Y, Binz J, Numerick MJ, et al. (2003) Hepatoprotection by the farsenoid X receptor agonist GW4064 in rat models of intra- and extrahepatic cholestasis. J Clin Invest 112:1678-87.
[17] Shefer S, Salen G, Nguyen L, et al. (1988) Competitive inhibition of bile acid synthesis by endogenous cholestanol and sitosterol in sitosterolemia with xanthomatosis: effect on cholesterol 7alpha-hydroxylase. J Clin Invest 82:1833-9.
[18] Yang C, McDonald JG, Patel A, et al. (2006) Sterol intermediates from cholesterol biosynthetic pathway as liver X receptor ligands. J Biol Chem 281:27816-26.
[19] Hąc-Wydroa K, Wydrob P, Jagodaa A, Kapusta J. (2007) The study on the interaction between phytosterols and phospholipids in model membranes. Chemistry and Physics of Lipids 150: 22-34.
[20] Fatemi, S.H., G.E. Cullan, G.M. Cullan, J.G. Sharp. (1985) Comparison of the intravenous and intraperitoneal routes of administration of tritiated thymidine in studies of cell production in the gastrointestinal tract of the rat. Virchows Archiv B Cell Pathology Zell-Patologie. 48:69-76.

6

How Do Lampreys Avoid Cholestasis After Bile Duct Degeneration?

Mayako Morii[1], Yoshihiro Mezaki[2], Kiwamu Yoshikawa[2], Mitsutaka Miura[2], Katsuyuki Imai[2], Taku Hebiguchi[1], Ryo Watanabe[1], Yoshihiro Asanuma[3], Hiroaki Yoshino[1] and Haruki Senoo[2]
Departments of [1]Pediatric Surgery
[2]Cell Biology and Morphology,
Akita University Graduate School of Medicine,
[3]Akita University School of Health Sciences
Japan

1. Introduction

Biliary atresia (BA) is the most common cause of cholestasis during infancy for which an etiology remains undetermined. Patients require hepatic portoenterostomy within the first 2-3 months of life in order to restore bile flow from the liver into the intestinal tract. Even with successful surgery, in most patients the disease advances to end-stage cirrhosis due to the progressive destruction of bile ducts, and requires liver transplantation in order for long term survival to be viable (Mack & Sokol, 2005). Without a better understanding of the etiology and pathogenesis of the progressive cholangitic mechanisms in BA, improvement in the prognosis of non-transplantation patients should not be expected. Despite the importance of understanding these underlying mechanisms, research of BA has been hindered by the lack of a suitable animal model.

The lamprey is the only vertebrate in which bile duct disappearance occurs spontaneously during metamorphosis. Multiple reports have described a histological similarity between human and lamprey bile duct loss and suggested that the lamprey be used as an animal model in the study of BA (Youson & Sidon, 1978; Boomer et al., 2010; Morii et al., 2010). While the lamprey differs greatly from humans in both appearance and character, striking parallels exist between the behavior of their hepatocytes and biliary epithelial cells. Understanding the mechanism that controls cholestasis in the lamprey liver during metamorphosis might contribute to the development of treatments for obstructive cholangiopathy in human BA.

2. Lamprey biology

The lampreys, which include 38 species, are considered the ancestral representatives of vertebrates, and studies regarding their genealogy, phylogeny and biology have all been made in detail (Hardisty & Potter, 1971).

2.1 Lamprey life cycle

All lampreys have a complex life cycle that consists of both larval and adults stages with a full metamorphosis in between. Eggs laid in freshwater streams hatch, giving rise to young larvae which burrow into the mud and feed on detritus. After a period of 4 to 7 years, larvae undergo metamorphosis into an adult lamprey.

Adult lampreys can be divided into two categories, parasitic (anadromous) and non-parasitic (fluvial), based on their adult life history immediately following metamorphosis. After metamorphosis, parasitic lampreys migrate to lakes or oceans in order to parasitize fish. After several years, sexually mature adults migrate back to freshwater streams to reproduce. Non-parasitic lampreys, on the other hand, stop feeding before the commencement of metamorphosis, spawn and die without ever resuming feeding.

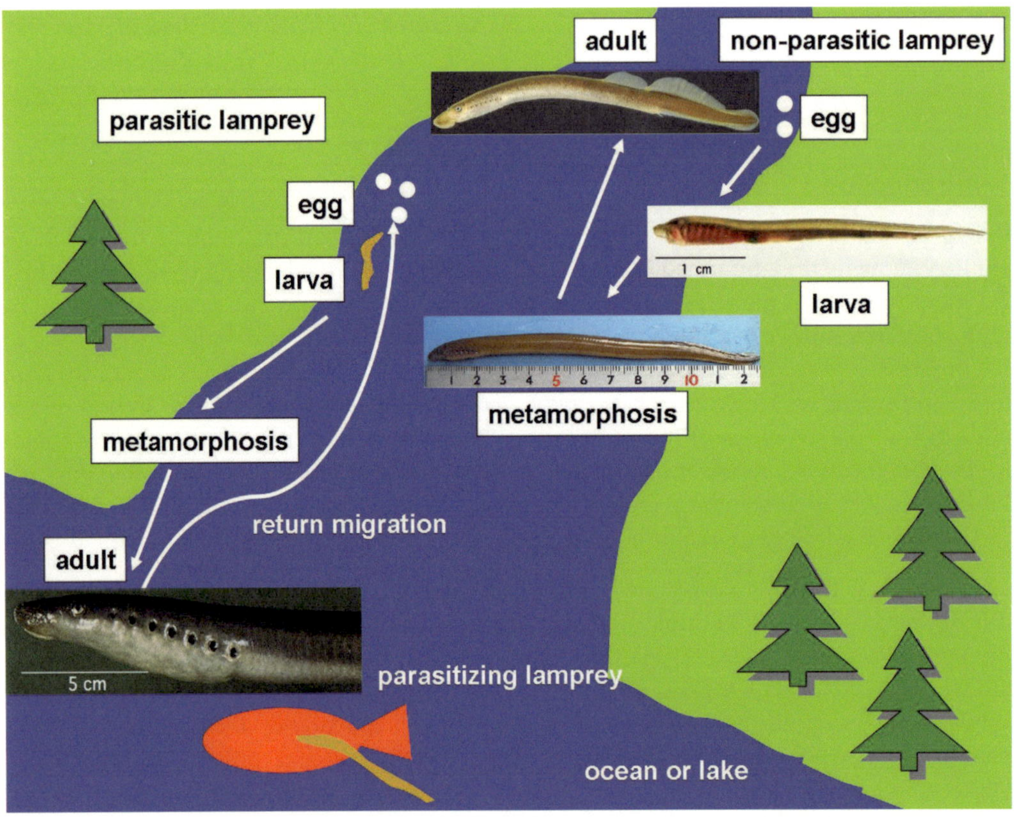

Fig. 1. Reproductive life cycle of lampreys.

Figure 1 illustrates the reproductive life cycle of lampreys with photographs taken during different stages of development. An undeveloped larva has no eyes, and the green bile juice of its gall bladder is visible through the abdominal skin. At the onset of metamorphosis, a small eye begins to appear. The top and bottom photographs show parasitic and non-parasitic adult lampreys, each with a prominent oral disc.

2.2 The lamprey in Japan

The occurrence of three *Lethnteron* species, *L. japonicum* (parasitic), *L. kessleri* (non-parasitic) and *L. reissneri* (non-parasitic), have been reported in Japan (Yamazaki & Goto, 1998). Taxonomically, these species are closely related to one another and may constitute a group of satellite species, a term used to describe ancestor-descendant pairs in lampreys. Morphological similarities between parasitic and non-parasitic species have supported evidence that different non-parasitic species evolved multiple times from parasitic species. Current hypotheses postulate that the evolution of non-parasitism in lampreys may be the result of a protracted larval stage (Yamazaki et al., 2001).

2.3 Metamorphosis of the lamprey

During metamorphosis, lampreys develop functional eyes and a prominent oral disk with teeth. Internal organs, such as the alimentary canal and the liver, also undergo significant changes during this process. A non-parasitic lamprey in Japan, *L. reissneri*, stops feeding prior to the commencement of metamorphosis and never resume feeding because major alterations to the digestive system, including loss of the gall bladder and biliary tree in the liver and prominent atrophy of the intestinal canal, have occurred. A parasitic lamprey in Japan, *L. japonicum*, parasitizes fish in order to feed on blood and tissue which is then digested by its potent saliva. This change in feeding behavior makes digestive requirements of the adult parasite much different than those of the larval stage lamprey. In order to accommodate these changes, bile ducts disappear entirely and the intestinal canal becomes specialized for nutrient absorption (Higashi et al., 2005).

2.4 Bile salts of lampreys

Bile salts are the major end-metabolites of cholesterol and serve an important function in digestion. For many species of fish, they are also used as potent olfactory stimulants. The increased use of cholesterol by vertebrates as compared to invertebrates is believed to have been the cause of a major evolutionary shift, allowing vertebrates to better regulate cell membrane fluidity, insulate nerve fibers and synthesize steroid hormones. The increased levels of cholesterol seen in vertebrates require tightly regulated systems for controlling the synthesis of cholesterol and its elimination from the body. The ability to remove cholesterol from the body in a regulated fashion is accomplished by the parallel development of a hepatobiliary tract.

Sea lampreys are known to produce, release or contain four kinds of sulfated bile salts (Fig. 2). Three kinds of bile salts (petromyzonol sulfate, petromyzonamine disulfate, and petromyzosterol disulfate) in particular are known to be produced by larval lampreys and excreted in feces so that they may function as migratory pheromones for adults (Fig. 2). 3-ketopetromyzonol sulfate, an oxidized analog of petromyzonol sulfate, is produced and released by sexually mature male sea lampreys, and functions as a sex pheromone that attracts ovulating females (Burns et al., 2011).

3. Hepatobiliary structure of larval lampreys

During the larval period, lampreys have a biliary system that is similar to that of humans. Bile acids are synthesized from cholesterol in hepatocytes and secreted into the alimentary

petromyzonol sulfate (X is α-OH)

3-ketopetromyzonol sulfate (X is =O)

petromyzonamine disulfate

petromyzosterol disulfate

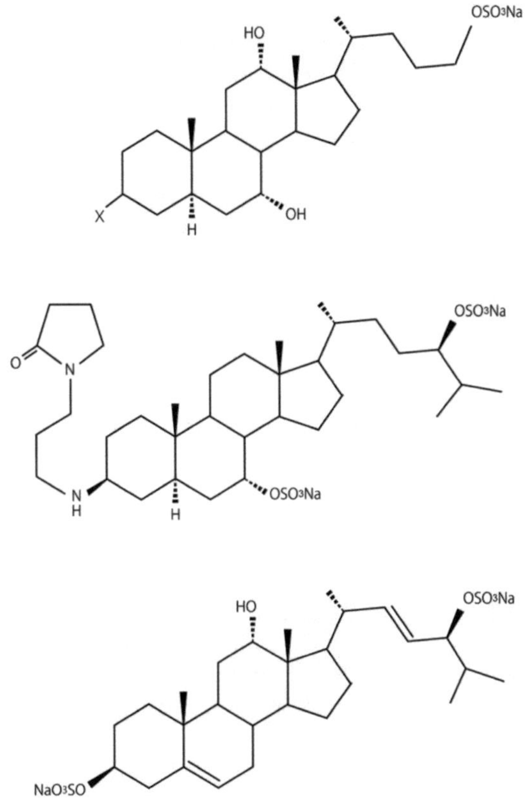

Fig. 2. Principal bile salts of the sea lamprey.

canal through the bile duct. We analyzed the morphology of *L. reissneri*, a non-parasitic lamprey, as they do not migrate, allowing larvae, metamorphosing animals and adults to be collected from the same waters (Yamazaki & Goto, 2000).

3.1 General liver structure of larval lampreys and humans

Larval lampreys have a complete biliary system similar to that of humans. The system contains terminal hepatic venules, a portal triad and sinusoids. The portal triad is composed of a portal vein, a hepatic artery and bile ducts and the interconnecting plates of hepatocytes which surround the sinusoidal channels run between the central vein and the portal triad. The entire liver appears fan-shaped and is similar to the functional unit in the human liver known as the acinus (Fig. 3).

3.2 Larval biliary system

Five-micron serial sections were made from the livers of larval lampreys and stained with hematoxylin and eosin (HE). Some slides were recorded digitally using NanoZoomer Digital Pathology (Hamamatsu Photonics, Hamamatsu, Japan). Studies of serial sections confirmed that larvae have a complete biliary system similar to that of humans (Fig. 4).

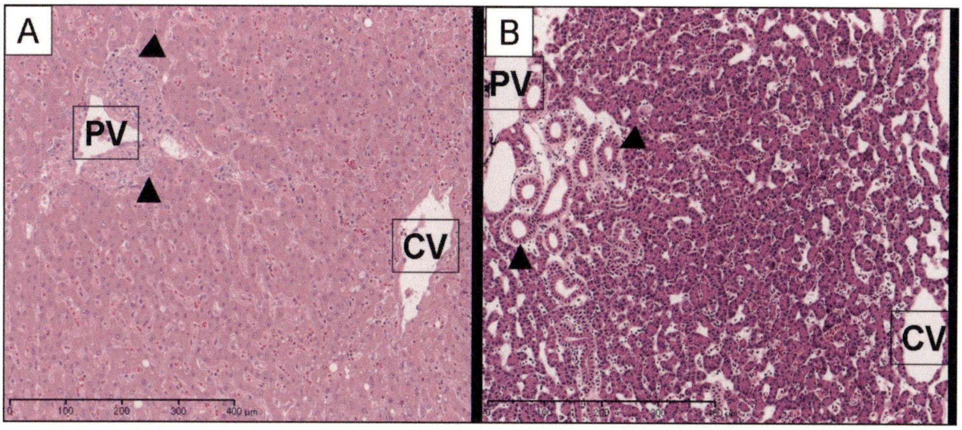

Fig. 3. Histologic analyses of human (panel A) and larval lamprey (panel B) liver specimens using HE staining to show the general liver architecture. PV: portal vein. CV: central vein (branch of hepatic vein). ▲: bile ducts.

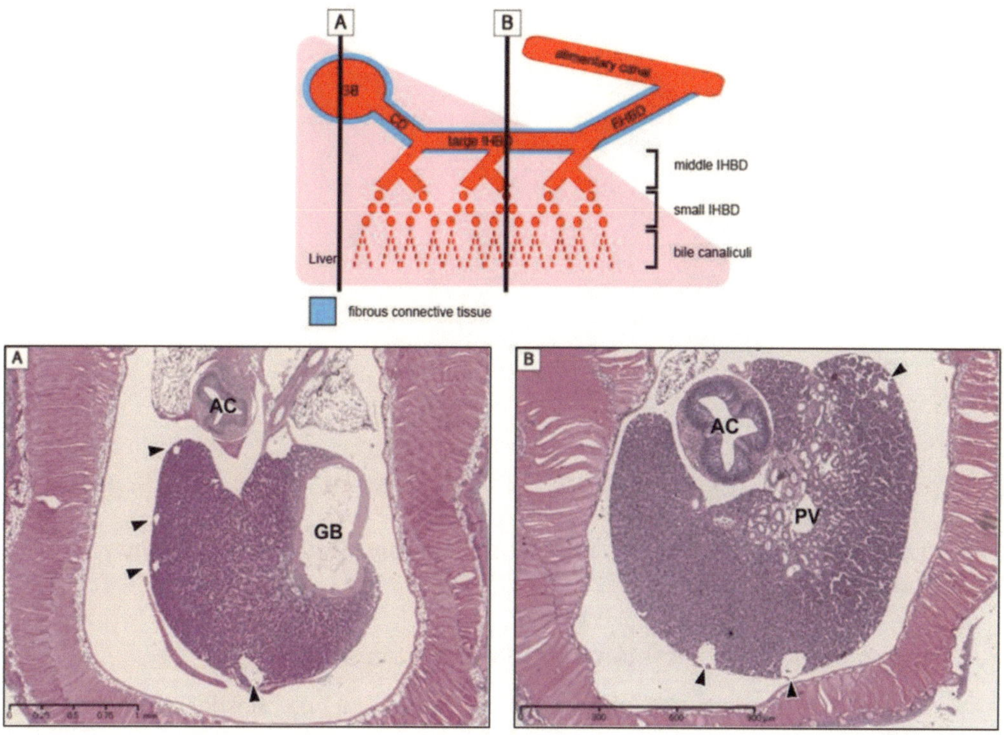

Fig. 4. Schematic diagram of the bile duct system in the liver of a lamprey larva and low-power micrographs of cross-sections taken at points A and B (depicted in panels A and B, respectively). GB: gallbladder. CD: cystic duct. EHBD: extrahepatic bile duct. IHBD: intrahepatic bile duct. AC: alimentary canal. PV: portal vein. ▲: hepatic veins.

The gall bladder (GB) was located at the cranial end and the cystic duct (CD) connected the GB to a large intra-hepatic bile duct (IHBD) that collected bile juice from the liver. The large

IHBD was composed of a simple columnar epithelium surrounded by some fibrous connective tissue. The middle IHBDs were also composed of simple columnar epithelia but they lacked surrounding connective tissue. The small IHBDs consisted of simple cuboidal epithelia. A cross-section of the central region of the liver revealed a single lobe with a large IHBD, portal vein and hepatic artery, as well as hepatic veins present at the edge.

3.3 Structure of bile canaliculi

Prior to examination by transmission electron microscopy (TEM), livers of larval lampreys were fixed in 2.5% glutaraldehyde in 0.1 M cacodylate buffer (pH 7.4) for 3 h, rinsed with the same buffer (pH 7.4), postfixed in 2% osmium tetroxide for 2 h, dehydrated and then embedded in Epon-812 resin. Ultrathin sections of the livers were cut at 60 nm by an ultramicrotome (LKB 250) and stained with uranylacetate and lead citrate. The stained sections were examined under a transmission electron microscope (JEM-1200EX, JEOL) at an acceleration voltage of 100 kV.

Electron microscopic analyses of specimens during the larval period revealed bile canaliculi within lumina surrounded by three to six hepatocytes. Numerous microvilli were present on the apical membrane of the canaliculi (Fig. 5).

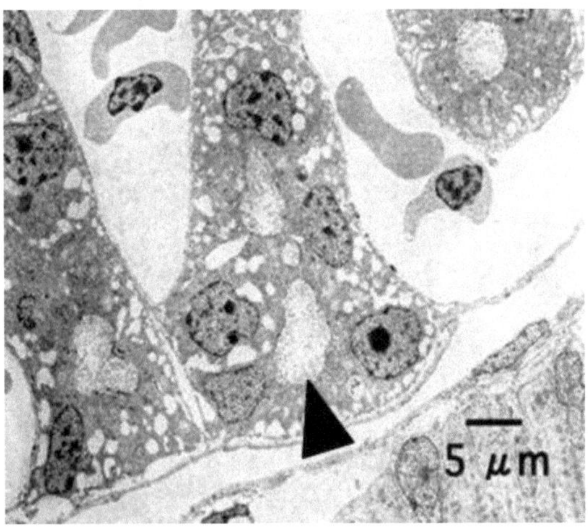

Fig. 5. Transmission electron micrograph of the bile canaliculi of a lamprey larva.
▲: bile canaliculus.

4. Changes in the biliary system at metamorphosis

As part of the normal ontogeny of the sea lamprey, the entire bile-transport apparatus of the larvae disappears completely during metamorphosis; however, the cause of this BA is not known.

Disappearance of the bile ducts accompanied by inflammatory change or necrosis have, until recently, been considered the primary processes occurring during human BA. Several recent studies have reported, however, that apoptosis of biliary epithelial cells takes place during BA (Sasaki et al., 2001; Harada et al., 2008; Funaki et al., 1998). Apoptosis, or programmed cell death, is defined in the narrow sense as the process associated with nucleic acid fragmentation due to a caspase cascade, which eventually leads to caspase-3 accumulation in the cell nucleus (Alnemri et al., 1996). Cleavage of DNA by caspase cascades can be induced by various factors in many kinds of cells. These factors can include viral infection in biliary epithelial cells, ischcemia in the neurocytes of prenatal fetuses, cholestasis in the hepatocytes with intestinal failure-associated liver diseases.

We have previously demonstrated that apoptosis plays a significant role in the degeneration of lamprey bile ducts during metamorphosis (Morii et al., 2010). The involvement of apoptosis in both human BA and lamprey bile duct degeneration during metamorphosis indicates that lampreys could be used as a model animal for studying the etiology and underlying mechanisms of human BA.

4.1 Liver structure in metamorphosing lampreys and humans with BA

The Liver structures of metamorphosing lamprey have some similarities to those of humans with BA at the time of hepatic portoenterostomy during the first 2-3 months of life.

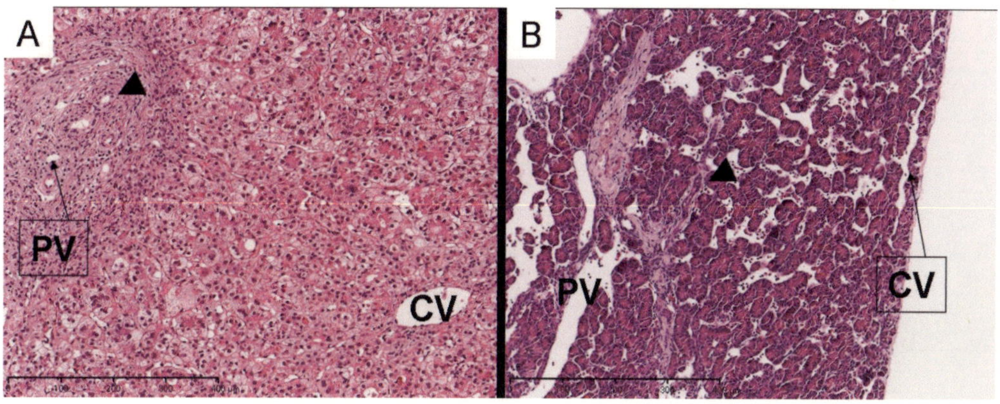

Fig. 6. Histological analyses of liver specimens from a human with BA (panel A) and a metamorphosing lamprey (panel B) using HE staining. The photograph in panel A was taken when the patient underwent initial surgery for treatment of BA. PV: portal vein. CV: central vein (branch of hepatic vein). ▲: bile ducts.

Both micrographs in figure 6 show the marked expansion of portal space with fibrous connective tissue and degeneration of bile ducts with intercanalicular bile stasis or debris. However, the intracellular bile stasis, proliferation of lobular bile ducts and infiltration of polymorphonuclear leukocytes are observed only in the human specimen (Fig. 6), indicating more severe cholestasis in human BA as compared to lamprey biliary degeneration.

4.2 Apoptosis of biliary epithelial cells

Five-micron serial sections of paraffin-embedded blocks were made from the livers of lampreys during the early metamorphosing stage. Alternate sections were stained with HE or apoptotic markers such as terminal deoxynucleotidyl transferase dUTP nick end labeling (TUNEL) or immunohistochemistry using an antibody against active caspase-3.

4.2.1 Light microscopy

Figure 7 shows the cross section of the GB stained with HE. The upper edge of the cross section is the mucosa of the GB, which is composed of biliary epithelial cells. The amount of fibrous connective tissue beneath the mucosa increases, and the biliary epithelial cells degenerates as the height of the epithelial cells is reduced. A muscular layer with myocytes was not present in the mucosa and some basophilic components were observed between the fibrils.

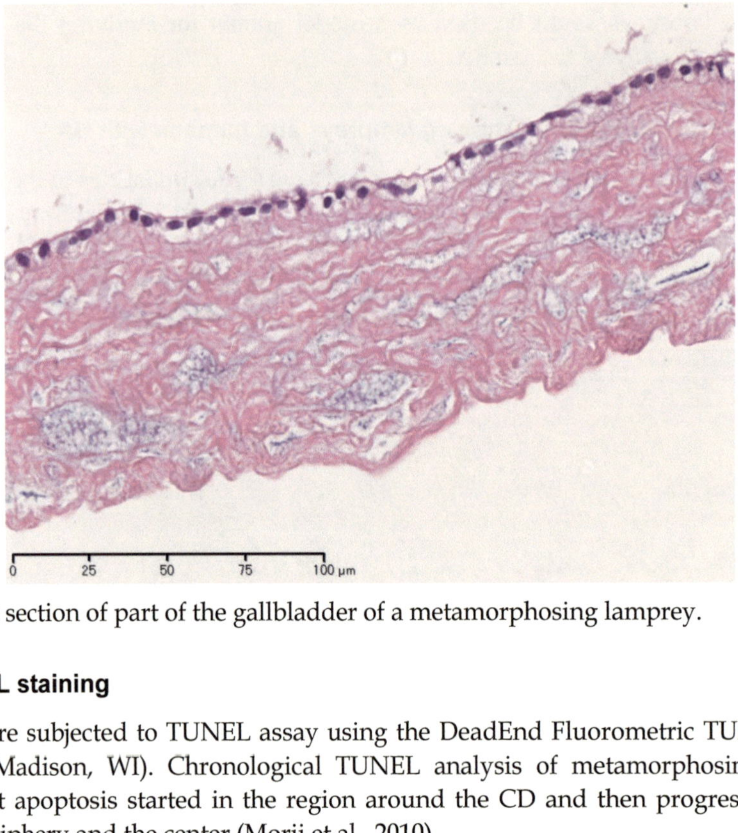

Fig. 7. Cross section of part of the gallbladder of a metamorphosing lamprey.

4.2.2 TUNEL staining

Sections were subjected to TUNEL assay using the DeadEnd Fluorometric TUNEL System (Promega, Madison, WI). Chronological TUNEL analysis of metamorphosing lampreys showed that apoptosis started in the region around the CD and then progressed towards both the periphery and the center (Morii et al., 2010).

Figure 8 shows that the epithelial cells of the GB were positive for TUNEL staining. TUNEL-positive staining was also observed within the extracellular debris among the connective tissue of the submucosa. This extracellular debris corresponded to the basophilic components seen in figure 7. In humans, apoptotic cells, which contain basophilic components such as nucleic acids, are processed and degraded promptly by phagocytosis. If intercellular components cannot be processed, the resulting autoimmune diseases lead to morbidity in humans. In lampreys, the activity of phagocytotic cells may not be sufficient for complete degradation of apoptotic cells, leading to the presence of the TUNEL-positive cell debris observed in the submucosa. In larval lampreys, we did not detect any signs of DNA fragmentation of the biliary system, which included hepatocytes, bile canaliculi, the extrahepatic and intrahepatic bile ducts, the CD and the GB (date not shown).

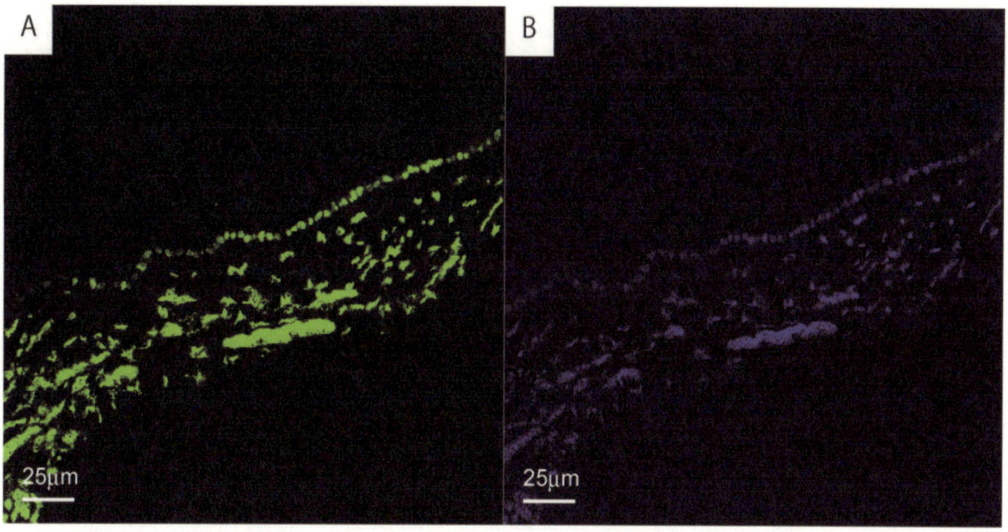

Fig. 8. TUNEL staining of the GB of a metamorphosing lamprey. The upper most layer is the mucosa epithelial cell layer. Most epithelial cells are TUNEL-positive (panel A, green). Nuclei are stained with TO-PRO-3 (panel B, blue).

4.2.3 Active caspase-3 staining

To confirm that these cells were undergoing apoptosis, cross sections of early metamorphosing stage lampreys were stained with an antibody against active caspase-3, a key regulator of the apoptotic cascade activated during the early phase of apoptosis prior to DNA fragmentation.

The deparaffinized sections were treated with 0.2% Triton X-100 in PBS for permeabilization, incubated with a blocking solution (1% bovine serum albumin), and then incubated with 1:50 rabbit anti-active caspase-3 antibody (Cell Signaling Technologies, Danvers, MA) at 4°C overnight. Following washes, the sections underwent incubation with 1:100 biotin SP-conjugated AffiniPure goat anti-rabbit IgG (Jackson ImmunoResearch, West Grove, PA). Finally, the sections were treated with 1:100 streptavidin, Alexa Fluor 488 conjugate (Invitrogen, Carlsbad, CA). Nuclei were stained with TO-PRO-3 (Invitrogen).

Caspase-3 has been identified as a key mediator of apoptosis. In response to various death signals, caspase-3 proenzyme is activated in the cytoplasm before it enters the nucleus, where it leads to the fragmentation of DNA (Woo et al., 1998; Zheng et al., 1998; Kamada et al., 2005).

In our observation, epithelial cells of the CD, GB and part of the large IHBD at the early metamorphosing stage were negative for active caspase-3 staining (data not shown) while they were positive for TUNEL staining, indicating the occurrence of more advanced apoptotic processes in these regions; however, the nuclei of the epithelial cells of middle IHBDs were positive for active caspase-3 staining (Fig. 9). Collectively, these observations indicate that apoptotic cascades in the CD, GB and the large IHBD precede those in the middle IHBDs.

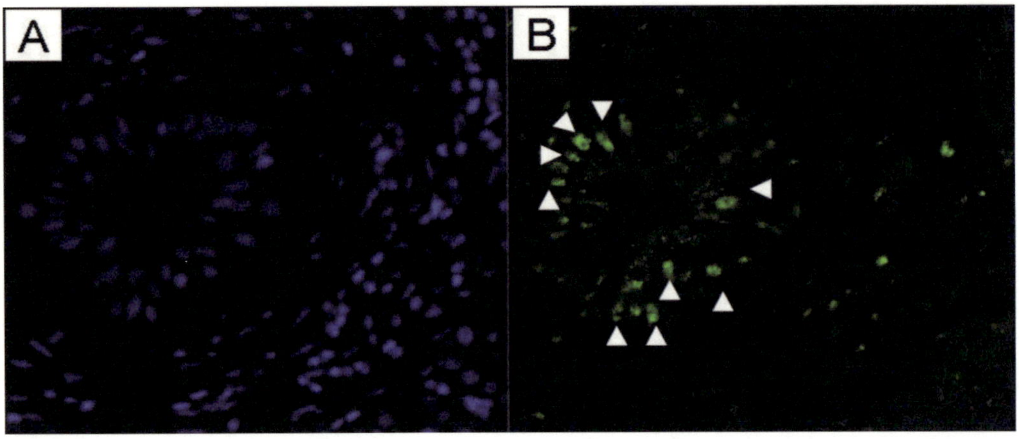

Fig. 9. Immunohistochemical staining of biliary epithelial cells of an early metamorphosing lamprey with an antibody against active caspase-3. The middle IHBDs of metamorphic lampreys were stained with an antibody against active caspase-3 (green, panel B), followed by staining with TO-PRO-3 (blue, panel A) for nuclei. Δ: nuclei of biliary epithelial cells.

4.2.4 Cross-reactivity of an antibody against human active caspase-3 to lamprey active caspase-3

In order to confirm the presence of caspase cascades in lampreys and the cross-reactivity of an antibody raised against human active caspase-3 to lamprey active caspase-3, a primary culture of lamprey cells was treated with staurosporine, an apoptosis-inducing reagent, and then analyzed in order to ascertain the expression of active caspase-3 using western blotting.

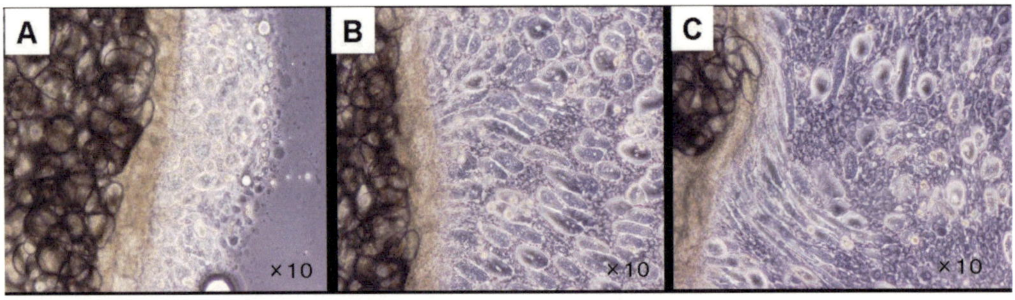

Fig. 10. Migration of cellular patches. Primary cell culture after 5 h (panel A), 24 h (panel B) and 2 days (panel C).

Anesthetized lampreys were washed with phosphate buffered saline (PBS) solution with 100 U/mL penicillin and 100 mg/mL streptomycin. The epidermis was then scraped off using an operating knife blade starting at the tail of lamprey. Scraped tissue was placed onto plastic dishes and cultured for 7 days in L-15 medium (Invitrogen) with 10% fetal bovine serum, 100 U/mL penicillin and 100 mg/mL streptomycin in a CO_2 ambient incubator at 20°C. Cellular patches were formed by the migration of tissue from small explants (Fig. 10). Culture medium was changed every 3 days. After 7 days of incubation, we removed the explants from tissue clumps. Cells reaching 30–60% confluence were harvested and washed with the medium and seeded onto new dishes.

Three days later, cells were treated by 1 μM staurosporine (Cosmo Bio, Tokyo, Japan) and collected after 4 h. After centrifugation at 1,000 x g for 5 min, the pellets were washed by PBS and dissolved in SDS gel-loading buffer. Two micrograms of cell pellets were separated by sodium dodecyl sulfate poly acrylamide gel electrophoresis (SDS-PAGE) and analyzed by Western-blotting using rabbit anti-active caspase-3 antibody (Cell signaling Technologies, Danvers, MA).

In mammals, pro-caspase-3, which is about 35 kD, is present in both mitochondria and the cytosol. When a death signal is transmitted to the cells, caspase cascades are activated, resulting in pro-caspase-3 dividing into two activated fragments. Activated fragments accumulate in cell nuclei, leading to nucleic acid fragmentation. The anti-active caspase-3 antibody we used can detect activated fragments of approximately 17 kD. Western blot analysis of lamprey cells from samples treated with staurosporine displayed a band of approximately 17 kD (Fig. 11) which was not present in untreated control cells, indicating that the band in treated cells corresponded to the presence of active caspase-3.

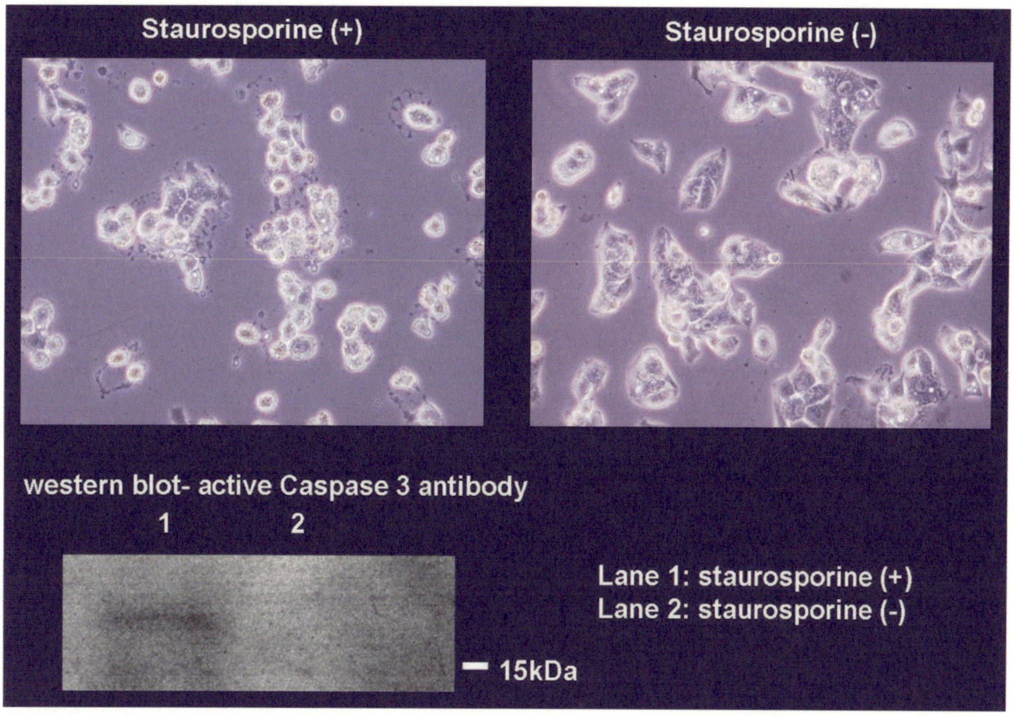

Fig. 11. Western blot analysis of untreated or staurosporine-treated lamprey cell.

4.2.5 Electron microscopy

TEM observation revealed apoptotic features in the biliary epithelial cells of metamorphosing lampreys.

The electron micrograph showed highly electron-dense materials and dispersed chromatin in the nucleus, and the cell surface was characterized by the loss of microvilli and the dome-shaped morphological appearance of the apical side (Fig. 12, panel A). Panel B shows a higher-magnification view of the apoptotic cell with chromatin condensation occurring at the periphery of the nuclear membrane.

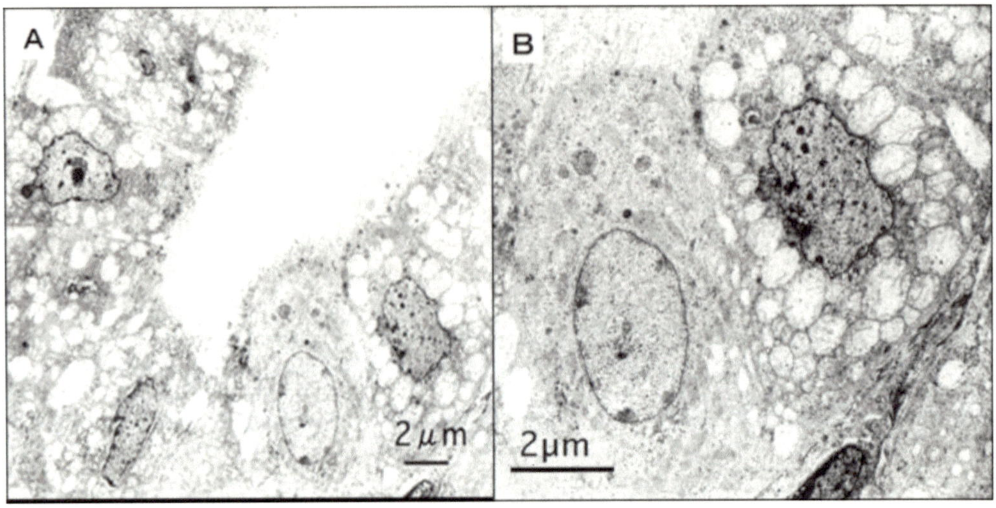

Fig. 12. Transmission electron micrograph of the middle IHBD of a metamorphosing lamprey. Lower right portion of panel A is magnified in panel B, showing characteristic features of apoptotic cells.

5. Biliary atresia in adult lampreys

While adult lampreys lacked a bile duct system, fibrous connective tissue remained at the porta hepatis. Electron microscopy also confirmed the absence of the interstitia between hepatocytes, known as bile canaliculi. Despite such obvious BA, lampreys do not develop either biliary cirrhosis or liver dysfunction.

5.1 Liver architecture of adult lampreys and humans with BA

Figure 13 shows micrographs of liver specimens from a human with BA at the time of liver transplantation (panel A) as well as an adult lamprey (panel B), both prepared using HE

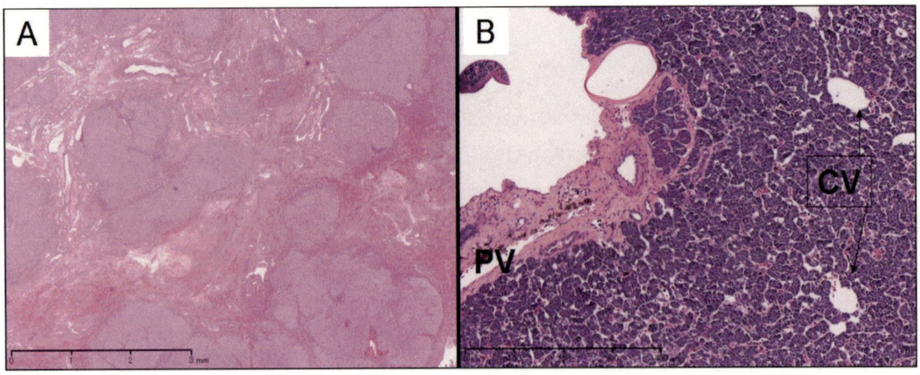

Fig. 13. Micrograph of the cirrhotic liver of a human with BA (panel A) and the liver of an adult lamprey (panel B).

staining. Despite the loss of all bile ducts in both specimens, the prognosis of each organism is much different. In the human specimen, there are nodules of regenerating hepatocytes, but their connections with the vascular supply and bile drainage system are destroyed. Irregular scarring caused by massive increases in fibrocollagenous tissue is also present.

In the adult lamprey specimen, the only remaining fibrous connective tissue can be found at the porta hepatis, and a complete absence of bile ducts can be noted. Some pigments that appear to be vestiges of bile stasis can be observed between the fibrils. The parenchymal cells appear undamaged and seem to keep blood supply abundant through sinusoidal connection.

5.2 Disappearance of bile canaliculi

In the adult lamprey specimen, neither bile canaliculi nor tight junctions between hepatocytes could be identified, even when electron microscopy was employed. Hepatocytes in adult lampreys showed a complete loss of their canalicular (apical) membrane (Fig. 14). As adult lampreys lose their entire biliary system including bile canaliculi during metamorphosis, bile acids, if they are synthesized in hepatocytes, must be released into circulation via the basolateral (sinusoidal) plasma membrane in order to serve as endocrine factors. Accumulation of lipid droplets was also observed, along with well-developed granular endoplasmic reticulum in the cytoplasm.

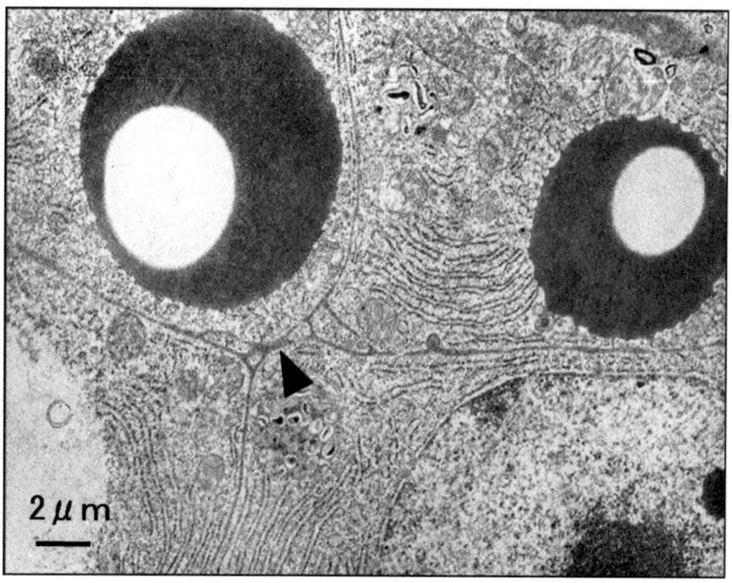

Fig. 14. Transmission electron micrograph of the absence of interstitia between hepatocytes (▲).

6. Cholesterol metabolism

In order to determine the organ in which they metabolize cholesterol, we intravenously injected adult male lampreys (*L. japonicum*) with ^{14}C-cholesterol and then radioassayed the liver, intestine, muscle, gonads (testis), and epidermis after periods of 1, 3 and 16 h had elapsed. As adult lampreys obtain cholesterol from the blood and tissue of fish on which they feed, they must have a means of metabolizing or accumulating cholesterol. Male lampreys must also use cholesterol in order to synthesize 3-Ketopetromyzonol sulfate for use as a sex pheromone in attracting ovulating females. We recorded levels of radioactivity in the liver and intestine that were approximately 10-times greater than those recorded in the muscle, gonads and epidermis at 3 h after injection. Radioactivity levels measured in the muscle, gonads and epidermis were saturated at 16 h post-injection. These findings indicate that ^{14}C-cholesterol did accumulate in these tissues; however, that radioactivity levels decreased in the liver and intestine in the period from 3 h to 16 h post-injection suggests that these tissues metabolized and eliminated some cholesterol over time.

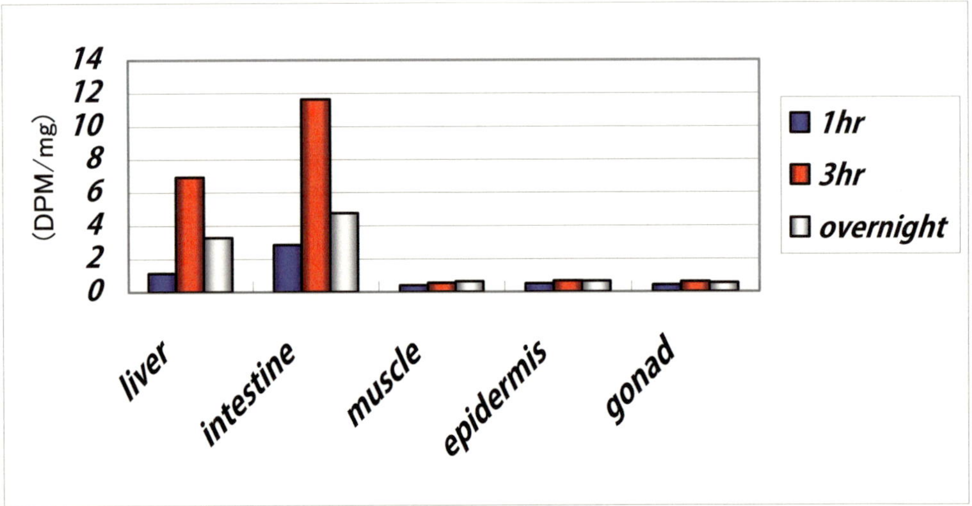

Fig. 15. Radioactivity detected in the liver and intestine was greater than that observed in the muscle, gonads and epidermis.

7. Discussion

Human BA can be categorized as either embryonic (fetal) or perinatal (acquired). The embryonic form of BA is believed to be caused by mutations in genes regulating biliary development and, while the etiology of the perinatal form of BA is not completely understood, proposed precipitating factors include viral infections, toxins, vascular and immune mediators (Mack & Sokol, 2005). If the initial surgery used to treat BA can successfully restore bile flow, treatment will still be complicated by progressive destruction of bile ducts resulting in ductopenia. BA in humans is not wholly distinguished by any single disorder during the perinatal period, it is also characterized by the slow and continuous degeneration of biliary epithelial cells. There is no doubt that this destruction of biliary epithelial cells plays a role in the inflammatory processes seen in livers affected by BA. Furthermore, recent studies have reported the occurrence of apoptosis in biliary epithelial cells of humans affected by BA (Sasaki et al., 2001; Harada et al., 2008; Funaki et al., 1998). Two potential causes of the progressive disappearance of biliary epithelial cells observed in human BA are purported: an autoimmune response induced by the initial disorder in the biliary epithelial cells, and cytotoxicity of the bile acids stasis. These two causes could potentially account for the common behaviors of hepatocytes and biliary epithelial cells in both human and lamprey livers.

Many previous studies have indicated a viral cause of BA, such as reovirus type 3, group C rotavirus, and cytomegalovirus; however, these viruses are not always detected in BA patients (Bangaru et al., 1980; Riepenhoff-Talty et al., 1996). Mack *et al.* proposed that bile duct infection or injury due to rotavirus infection could be inciting factors leading to progressive, autoimmune-mediated damage of the biliary tree after recovery from infection (Mack & Sokol, 2005; Barnes et al., 2009). Incidentally, it has been revealed that programmed cell death in amphibian metamorphosis is induced by a selective auto-immune response, and that the immune system may contribute to the remodeling processes in vertebrate morphogenesis, universally (Mukaigasa et al., 2009). The onset of human BA always occurs during the pre-natal or perinatal periods despite the fact that rotavirus infection with acholic stool and other viral infections are so common among preschool children and infants under one year of age. It is likely that humans are sensitive to the inducement of apoptosis during pre-natal or perinatal periods in which the fetus loses many prenatal structures such as the ductus arteriosus, ductus venosus, webbing between the fingers, and branchial arches. The suppression of autoimmune-mediated apoptosis could be a valuable tool in the treatment of human BA.

Generally, bile salts are synthesized through a many-stepped process starting with cholesterol oxidation and will damage the liver if they are not correctly discharged. The main mechanism of maintaining cholesterol homeostasis in many vertebrates is the enterohepatic circulation, the obstruction of which is fatal due to the cytotoxicity of bile. The adult lamprey, however, loses its entire bile duct system without developing the pathological effects of cholestasis. It was confirmed that the lamprey metabolized cholesterol into bile alcohol within the liver and intestinal canal despite the loss of bile canaliculi in the hepatocytes, which resulted in the loss of the apical membrane used for bile secretion. These results indicate that 3-ketopetromyzonol sulfate, a bile alcohol produced in the adult male lamprey, is probably released into circulation via the basolateral (sinusoidal) plasma membrane. Sulfation is an important metabolic pathway responsible for the detoxification and elimination of bile acids in many species such as hamsters, monkeys, guinea pigs and humans. Sulfated bile acids are less toxic to cells than those without a sulfate group. The sulfation of bile acids also increases their solubility, enhancing their ability to be released into the circulation by ATP-binding cassette transporters via the basolateral (sinusoidal) plasma membrane and to be excreted in urine, especially under cholestatic conditions. Sulfation plays an important role in maintaining bile acid homeostasis under pathologic conditions in mammals. The proportion of sulfated bile acids differs markedly between species, and is very small in humans (Alnouti, 2009). In mammals, the sulfation of bile acids and the expression of the ATP-binding cassette transporters of the basolateral plasma membrane, such as multidrug resistance-associated protein 3 and multidrug resistance-associated protein 4, are regulated by nuclear receptors, such as farnesoid X receptor, for which bile acids are known to be a ligand.

It is still unclear which process occurs first in the metamorphosing lamprey liver, cessation of the synthesis of larval bile alcohols by the hepatocytes or apoptosis of the biliary epithelial cells. The stage by stage features of hepatocyte transformation with a gradual loss of bile canaliculi (Sidon & Youson, 1983) along with the gradual disappearance of tight junctions at the bile canaliculi and an increase in area occupied by gap junctions (Youson et al., 1987) have been described in previous studies. Moreover, the degeneration of bile ducts has been associated with the development of marked periductal fibrosis due to fibroblast activation caused by leaked biliary materials (Youson et al., 1987; Yamamoto et al., 1986). Our observation of apoptosis in biliary epithelial cells detected prior to changes in hepatocyte morphology (Morii et al., 2010) was consistent with the results of previous reports. Intrahepatic cholestasis may regulate the remodeling of hepatocytes by changing the way cholesterol is metabolized, the expression of transporters in the basolateral membrane and the disappearance of tight junctions in hepatocytes surrounding bile canaliculi. Understanding the means by which adult lampreys are able to avoid cholestasis without bile ducts could allow for valuable progress in the treatment of human obstructive cholangiopathy to be made.

8. Conclusions

Lampreys could serve as animal models in the study of cholestasis in humans. Understanding the mechanism that controls bile acid sulfation and the progress of apoptosis in biliary epithelial cells in the lamprey liver during BA could contribute to the development of treatment for obstructive cholangiopathy in humans. Unfortunately, as the molecular biology of the lamprey has not been well studied, these mechanisms have not yet been elucidated.

9. Acknowledgment

We would like to thank Dr. Hideki Sugiyama (Akita Prefectural Fisheries Promotion Center, Akita, Japan) and Mr. Masayuki Kumagai (Ziban Kankyo Consultant, Akita, Japan) for collecting and photographing lampreys, and for their helpful comments.

10. References

Alnemri, E. S., Livingston, D. J., Nicholson, D. W., Salvesen, G., Thornberry, N. A., Wong, W. W. & Yuan, J. (1996) Human ICE/CED-3 protease nomenclature. *Cell,* 87, 171, 0092-8674

Alnouti, Y. (2009) Bile Acid sulfation: a pathway of bile acid elimination and detoxification. *Toxicol Sci,* 108, 225-246, 1096-0929

Bangaru, B., Morecki, R., Glaser, J. H., Gartner, L. M. & Horwitz, M. S. (1980) Comparative studies of biliary atresia in the human newborn and reovirus-induced cholangitis in weanling mice. *Lab Invest,* 43, 456-462, 0023-6837

Barnes, B. H., Tucker, R. M., Wehrmann, F., Mack, D. G., Ueno, Y. & Mack, C. L. (2009) Cholangiocytes as immune modulators in rotavirus-induced murine biliary atresia. *Liver Int,* 29, 1253-1261, 1478-3231

Boomer, L. A., Bellister, S. A., Stephenson, L. L., Hillyard, S. D., Khoury, J. D., Youson, J. H. & Gosche, J. R. (2010) Cholangiocyte apoptosis is an early event during induced metamorphosis in the sea lamprey, Petromyzon marinus L. *J Pediatr Surg,* 45, 114-120, 0022-3468

Burns, A. C., Sorensen, P. W. & Hoye, T. R. (2011) Synthesis and olfactory activity of unnatural, sulfated 5beta-bile acid derivatives in the sea lamprey (Petromyzon marinus). *Steroids,* 76, 291-300, 0039-128X

Funaki, N., Sasano, H., Shizawa, S., Nio, M., Iwami, D., Ohi, R. & Nagura, H. (1998) Apoptosis and cell proliferation in biliary atresia. *J Pathol,* 186, 429-433, 0022-3417

Harada, K., Sato, Y., Isse, K., Ikeda, H. & Nakanuma, Y. (2008) Induction of innate immune response and absence of subsequent tolerance to dsRNA in biliary epithelial cells relate to the pathogenesis of biliary atresia. *Liver Int,* 28, 614-621, 1478-3223

Hardisty, M. W. & Potter, I. C. 1971. *The biology of lampreys.* London, New York,: Academic Press.

Higashi, N., Wake, K., Sato, M., Kojima, N., Imai, K. & Senoo, H. (2005) Degradation of extracellular matrix by extrahepatic stellate cells in the intestine of the lamprey, Lampetra japonica. *Anat Rec A Discov Mol Cell Evol Biol,* 285, 668-675, 1552-4884

Mack, C. L. & Sokol, R. J. (2005) Unraveling the pathogenesis and etiology of biliary atresia. *Pediatr Res,* 57, 87R-94R, 0031-3998

Morii, M., Mezaki, Y., Yamaguchi, N., Yoshikawa, K., Miura, M., Imai, K., Yoshino, H., Hebiguchi, T. & Senoo, H. (2010) Onset of apoptosis in the cystic duct during metamorphosis of a Japanese lamprey, Lethenteron reissneri. *Anat Rec (Hoboken),* 293, 1155-1166, 1932-8486

Mukaigasa, K., Hanasaki, A., Maeno, M., Fujii, H., Hayashida, S., Itoh, M., Kobayashi, M., Tochinai, S., Hatta, M., Iwabuchi, K., Taira, M., Onoe, K. & Izutsu, Y. (2009) The keratin-related Ouroboros proteins function as immune antigens mediating tail regression in Xenopus metamorphosis. *Proc Natl Acad Sci U S A,* 106, 18309-18314, 0027-8424

Riepenhoff-Talty, M., Gouvea, V., Evans, M. J., Svensson, L., Hoffenberg, E., Sokol, R. J., Uhnoo, I., Greenberg, S. J., Schakel, K., Zhaori, G., Fitzgerald, J., Chong, S., el-Yousef, M., Nemeth, A., Brown, M., Piccoli, D., Hyams, J., Ruffin, D. & Rossi, T. (1996) Detection of group C rotavirus in infants with extrahepatic biliary atresia. *J Infect Dis,* 174, 8-15, 0022-1899

Sasaki, H., Nio, M., Iwami, D., Funaki, N., Sano, N., Ohi, R. & Sasano, H. (2001) E-cadherin, alpha-catenin and beta-catenin in biliary atresia: correlation with apoptosis and cell cycle. *Pathol Int,* 51, 923-932, 1320-5463

Sidon, E. W. & Youson, J. H. (1983) Morphological changes in the liver of the sea lamprey, Petromyzon marinus L., during metamorphosis. II. Canalicular degeneration and transformation of the hepatocytes. *J Morphol,* 178, 225-246, 0022-2887

Yamamoto, K., Sargent, P. A., Fisher, M. M. & Youson, J. H. (1986) Periductal fibrosis and lipocytes (fat-storing cells or Ito cells) during biliary atresia in the lamprey. *Hepatology,* 6, 54-59, 0270-9139

Yamazaki, Y. & Goto, A. (1998) Genetic structure and differentiation of four Lethenteron taxa from the Far East, deduced from allozyme analysis. *Environmental Biology of Fishes,* 52, 149-161, 03781909

Yamazaki, Y. & Goto, A. (2000) Breeding season and nesting assemblages in two forms of Lethenteron reissneri, with reference to reproductive isolating mechanisms. *Ichthyological Research,* 47, 271-276, 13418998

Yamazaki, Y., Nagai, T., Iwata, A. & Goto, A. (2001) Histological comparisons of intestines in parasitic and nonparasitic lampreys, with reference to the speciation hypothesis. *Zoological Science,* 18, 1129-1134, 02890003

Youson, J. H., Ellis, L. C., Ogilvie, D. & Shivers, R. R. (1987) Gap junctions and zonulae occludentes of hepatocytes during biliary atresia in the lamprey. *Tissue Cell,* 19, 531-548, 0040-8166

Youson, J. H. & Sidon, E. W. (1978) Lamprey biliary atresia: first model system for the human condition? *Experientia,* 34, 1084-1086, 0014-4754